CIGARETTES, NICOTINE, & Health

Behavioral Medicine and Health Psychology Series

SERIES EDITOR
J. Rick Turner
HealthComm Consulting

Behavioral Medicine and Health Psychology brings the latest advances in these fields directly into undergraduate, graduate, and professional classrooms via individual texts that each present one topic in a self-contained manner. The texts also allow health professionals specializing in one field to become familiar with another by reading the appropriate volume, a task facilitated by their short length and their scholarly yet accessible format.

The development of the series is guided by its Editorial Board, which comprises experts from the disciplines of experimental and clinical psychology, medicine and preventive medicine, psychiatry and behavioral sciences, nursing, public health, biobehavioral health, behavioral health sciences, and behavioral genetics. Board members are based in North America, Europe, and Australia, thereby providing a truly international perspective on current research and clinical practice in behavioral medicine and health psychology.

Books in This Series

Stress & Health: Biological and Psychological Interactions
by William R. Lovallo

Understanding Caffeine: A Biobehavioral Analysis
by Jack E. James

Physical Activity and Behavioral Medicine
by James F. Sallis and Neville Owen

Behavior Change and Public Health in the Developing World
by John P. Elder

Cigarettes, Nicotine, and Health: A Biobehavioral Approach
by Lynn T. Kozlowski, Jack E. Henningfield, and Janet Brigham

CIGARETTES, NICOTINE, & Health

A Biobehavioral Approach

Lynn T. Kozlowski
Jack E. Henningfield · Janet Brigham

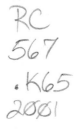
SAGE Publications
International Educational and Professional Publisher
Thousand Oaks   London   New Delhi

For information:

Sage Publications, Inc.
2455 Teller Road
Thousand Oaks, California 91320
E-mail: order@sagepub.com

Sage Publications Ltd.
6 Bonhill Street
London EC2A 4PU
United Kingdom

Sage Publications India Pvt. Ltd.
M-32 Market
Greater Kailash I
New Delhi 110 048 India

Printed in the United States of America

Library of Congress Cataloging-in-Publication Data

Kozlowski, Lynn T.
    Cigarettes, nicotine, and health : A biobehavioral approach / by
Lynn T. Kozlowski, Jack E. Henningfield, Janet Brigham.
        p. cm. — (Behavioral medicine and health psychology series ; v, 5)
    Includes index.
    ISBN 0-8039-5947-8 (alk. paper) — ISBN 0-0839-5946-X (alk. cloth)
    1. Tobacco—Physiological aspects. 2. Tobacco—Psychological aspects.
    3. Nicotine—Physiological aspects. 4. Health psychology.
    I. Henningfield, Jack E.
    II. Brigham, Janet. III. Title. IV. Series.
    RC567 .K65 2000
    616.86'5071—dc21   0-012631

01   02   03   04   05   06   10   9   8   7   6   5   4   3   2   1

Acquiring Editor: Jim Brace-Thompson
Production Editor: Claudia A. Hoffman
Editorial Assistant: Candice Crosetti
Typesetter: Marion Warren
Cover Designer: Michelle Lee

Contents

Series Editor's Introduction

Cigarettes, Nicotine, and Health: A Biobehavioral Approach, the fifth volume in this series, addresses worldwide tobacco use and its health consequences from a multidisciplinary perspective. Cigarette smoking, the most common form of tobacco use in many regions of the world, has enormous relevance for health promotion and disease prevention since it is the largest preventable cause of disability and death in many industrialized nations and a disturbingly accelerating trend in developing countries.

Professor Kozlowski has been a member of the Editorial Board since the inception of the series. He has now recruited two colleagues, Dr. Jack Henningfield and Dr. Janet Brigham, to coauthor this volume. All three scientists are exceptionally well qualified to introduce the reader to the many aspects (behavioral, biological, economic, public health) of cigarette marketing, use, and research.

As you will learn from the following chapters, a cigarette is an extremely sophisticated drug delivery system. The drug in question is nicotine (named after Jean Nicot, a French ambassador to Portugal in the 1500s). Nicotine is a psychoactive, addictive drug that is 10 times more potent, milligram for milligram, than cocaine and morphine. When cigarette smoke is inhaled into the lungs, nicotine is distributed throughout the body. In the brain, nicotine has many effects, including the stimulation of reward pathways.

However, the health consequences of tobacco use are devastating. For example, smokers may suffer from cardiovascular disease, cancer (especially, but not only, lung cancer), emphysema, and bronchitis. These diseases often lead not only to premature death but also to years of ill heath beforehand. Smoking can also cause or exacerbate musculoskeletal injuries and arthritis, and lead to birth defects. The combination of the severity of these conditions and the staggering numbers of individuals affected makes smoking reduction a major focus of the world's leading medical and public health authorities.

My thanks are extended to the authors for writing this volume, which illuminates a central topic in the fields of behavioral medicine and health psychology. Their organizational focus on cigarettes, nicotine, and health enables them to present a wide array of information on the consequences of tobacco use in a highly structured and integrated manner, and their insights complement their factual presentation very effectively.

—J. Rick Turner
Chapel Hill, North Carolina

Acknowledgments

Thanks to Richard O'Connor, Andrew Strasser, and Kristy Minarsky for critical readings of the manuscript. Thanks to J. Rick Turner, series editor, for his encouragement. In addition, Richard O'Connor and Andrew Strasser helped with references and manuscript preparation. Lisa Grove, Kathy Barefoot, and Virginia Lucas also helped prepare the manuscript.

1

Why *Biobehavioral?*
Why *Cigarettes, Nicotine,* and *Health?*

▶ *Rain. Mud. Cold. The night before the battle, the soldiers warm and brace themselves by smoking hand-rolled cigarettes. They inhale and hold their breath as long as they can. The steam from their breath mixes with the smoke they exhale in the night air. Thoughts travel away from the front. The soldiers dream of home. The cigarettes help them have some last easy moments to themselves.*

▶ *Happy Hour at the lounge. The slim young woman in a black sweater lights a long, thin cigarette. She has been smoking for years and handles the cigarette with elegant ease. She stacks her lighter neatly on the side of her pastel cigarette pack. She is with friends after work. Her friends, themselves smokers, are smoking along with her, matching her, cigarette for cigarette. They talk as they drink oversized glasses of wine. They smoke, unwind, and relax, talking over their plans for the evening.*

▶ *The man is opening his eyes. He is stretched out in bed. The coffeepot has an automatic timer. The smell of fresh coffee fills the bed-*

room. He reaches for a cigarette, carefully set out on his nightstand next to the ashtray, and lights it. He could find this cigarette in his sleep. He inhales the smoke deeply. He feels lightheaded. His brain seems to float in his head. He feels awake enough now to get up and pour himself some coffee.

▶ *The woman looks elderly. Her face is sunken and gray. Her skin hangs on her skeleton like an oversized suit. She is still in nightclothes in the late afternoon. One bony hand holds a cigarette to a surgical hole in her windpipe, and the other hand pumps at her belly to work her chest like a bellows. She knows that the laryngeal cancer will kill her. She is only 52.*

▶ *The plump girl, about 12, steals a full pack of her mother's cigarettes. The girl's short brown hair is spiked with blue. Her skin is as pale as a vampire's. Her lips are as red as dead roses. She has a silver ring in her nose. She practices smoking in front of her mirror. She purses her lips as if whistling and tries repeatedly to blow smoke rings in the light of two large candles. She studies her every move from many angles.*

▶ *The coworkers are huddled in the doorway to the office building. It is snowing, and they are trying to take as much shelter as they can at the sides of the big entry doors. One has put on an overcoat. The others have lifted up the collars of their suits and are holding their suits close around their necks. They are smoking, puffing rapidly, going through their cigarettes as fast as they can.*

▶ *From the deck of the ocean liner anchored offshore, moonlight reflects off the smooth waves. The man and woman kiss. He puts two cigarettes in his mouth, cups his hand over them, lights them, and hands one to her. Looking into his eyes, she puts her lips where his had been and draws in a long puff.*

▶ *The teenage boys hang out at the back entrance of the mall and ask young men to buy them beer. They can no longer smoke inside. They look tough—they want to look tough. They all smoke. They blow a curtain of smoke around them, perhaps to ward off strangers who might walk too close to their turf.*

▶ *The young parents are smoking in the worn-out living room. They have a small apartment. They are no longer permitted to smoke at work in the factory. Between them and the television is their baby's playpen. Smoke collects in the small room. The baby is shrieking loudly, pulling at her ear. This is her fifth ear infection in as many months. The parents are frustrated and annoyed, drawing in deeply and puffing out smoke in long sighs.*

▶ *The singer-songwriter is an artistically sad young man with a sparse blond beard. His hair is straight and plainly combed to frame his open face. He is weary from his real or invented pain and obviously bored with the television interview he is doing. He rubs his eyes. His eyes have huge shadows. Smoke from the cigarette he holds below his face rises into the camera's view.*

The scenes above sample the imagery of cigarette smoking: some appealing images, some unappealing, some mixed. They also provide examples of the *biobehavioral* realities of smoking, or those aspects of tobacco use that link the biology of tobacco's effects with the behavioral patterns in which people use it. When smokers inhale smoke into their lungs, they take the drug nicotine into their bodies and brains, where it affects how the smokers feel and act. When smokers display their cigarettes, they are saying something symbolic and personal about themselves. And when smokers smoke, they put themselves at risk, often knowingly, of early disability or death. This introductory chapter describes what is meant by a biobehavioral approach and explains why the topics of *cigarettes, nicotine,* and *health* are key organizing principles for this book on tobacco use and health.

▪ A Biobehavioral Approach

Figure 1.1 shows a schematic picture of what is involved in a biobehavioral approach. *Behavioral* issues refer to a broad class of factors that can influence behavior. In Figure 1.1, behavioral factors (e.g., culture, beliefs, thoughts, economics, or laws) can come from the top down to contribute to specific behaviors such

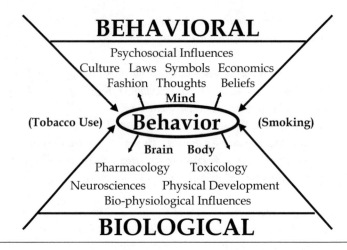

Figure 1.1. A Biobehavioral Model of Cigarette Smoking and Tobacco Use

as cigarette smoking. From the bottom up, *biological* factors (e.g., a person's age, genetics, or drug receptors in the brain) can also contribute to an overt behavior such as smoking a cigarette. The arrows move from the biological and the behavioral realms to influence what might be called *simple behaviors.* (The word *behavioral* refers here to the broad class of nonbiological influences, whereas *behavior* refers to the action being studied. Similarly, the word *biological,* as implied by the prefix *bio,* refers to a broader class of factors that reflect the physiology and anatomy of an organism's bodily functioning.) Simple behaviors, in turn, can have their own effects on both the behavioral and biological domains. If a behavior causes lung cancer and early death, it has a dramatic effect on the biological domain. If a behavior makes one perceive himself or herself either as a member of a group or as an outcast, it can have a significant effect on the behavioral domain.

Tobacco use and its relationship to health are best and most simply studied as a complex biobehavioral issue, as shown in Figure 1.1. The *bio* in biobehavioral refers to the complex array of biological and physiological forces involved with human life. Drugs (pharmacological or chemical agents) influence the workings of the body. Chemicals can also be poisons that damage health. *Toxicology* is the study of the disabilities and diseases caused by drugs. Drug taking, however, is a behavior, an action, or an act. Behavioral sciences are concerned with understanding behavior.

Although theoretically one might be able to analyze much, if not most, behavior in terms of underlying biological principles, in practice, science is at the present time far from being able to do so. Biobehavioral approaches provide a convenient, but not foolproof, way of breaking down complex, interdisciplinary problems. For example, within behavioral factors are these diverse elements:

- Words (e.g., calling someone a pejorative name)
- Culture (e.g., growing up on a tobacco farm when tobacco was a proud symbol of wealth, power, and pleasure)
- Beliefs (e.g., a conviction that people have a right to smoke or, alternatively, that smoking is sinful)
- Thoughts
- Laws (e.g., smoking restrictions)
- Perception of health risks

Consider the example of the stylish young woman in black who is smoking with her friends in the wine bar. Biological forces—a physical dependence on nicotine, the actions of nicotine on the brain—may be supporting her smoking, but behavioral forces can also be supporting her smoking. She may be smoking more than usual because of the social pressures of her friends' smoking (compare Kozlowski & Herman, 1984).

A biobehavioral approach has three basic elements. First, the approach is fundamentally interdisciplinary or multidisciplinary. Second, a simplifying distinction is made between the biological and nonbiological domains, or the behavioral and nonbehavioral domains (which is to say, the biological vs. the behavioral determinants). Third, the biobehavioral approach values studies more greatly if they include consideration of both biological and psychosocial influences on the behavior being studied.

Such an approach is needed to adequately study cigarettes, nicotine, and health. The study of this topic benefits from some grounding in principles of social psychology, cognitive psychology, behavioral pharmacology, pharmacology, physiology, epidemiology, medicine, and public health. Chapters throughout the book vary in their disciplinary emphases, but overall they orient the reader to an interdisciplinary, biobehavioral framework. Cigarette smoking is a complex problem, involving both chemical and nonchemical factors. The tobacco industry and society itself foster smoking and enable it to be sustained at high levels.

In this regard, cigarettes are of particular interest because they are (a) the most popular form of tobacco used in most areas of the world, (b) the most addictive form of tobacco used, and (c) the most deadly form of tobacco used. Cigarettes are also the objects we see. They are marketed and sold. They are what is displayed by smokers. They are what is consumed in the behavior of smoking. When one person sees another person smoking, it is the cigarette that is visible. The ingestion of nicotine itself is not easily visible, yet it is responsible for the dependence that develops to cigarette smoking. It is crucial to know something about the design, manufacture, and structure of cigarettes to understand details of how they are smoked. The modern cigarette has been designed carefully and specifically to maximize the effects smokers feel and the potential for becoming addicted to nicotine. The book also discusses other forms of tobacco, including smokeless tobacco, cigars, and pipes. These other forms of tobacco are at times popular and at other times almost never seen. Because they are sometimes popular, they are also worth our mention and concern.

▓ Nicotine

Nicotine is the chemical responsible for the drug pleasures of smoking. It is the chemical molecule that links the brain and body to the cigarette. No form of tobacco has been widely popular unless it delivers significant doses of nicotine to the brains of tobacco users (Kozlowski, 1982). Nicotine is a chemical with powerful actions that complicate and subvert the presumed free choice of people to smoke or not.

Nicotine Delivery Devices

Even if cigarettes and nicotine were merely addictive, they would still be of interest to those interested in the study of human motivation, or the inquiry into why human beings do what they do. We would wonder why smokers pay so much for cigarettes, why cigarettes sometimes appear to calm smokers down and at other times appear to stimulate or energize them. We would also ponder the prevalence of smoking in spite of the widespread death and disability that indicate that smoking is the world's most pressing public health problem. Health authorities around the world are trying to find ways to motivate tobacco users to stop, and to prevent nonusers from starting.

▨ Overview of the Rest of the Book

The world's scientific literature has become huge and is still growing rapidly. This small book omits a great deal of important work by important scholars. We have had to be very selective, and, understandably, we often emphasize what we have learned directly from our own research work. In addition to reporting "the facts," we believe that it is also important for professors to "profess" from time to time and offer some speculation on how the facts best fit together.

Chapter 2: The History of Nicotine Use

For millennia, nicotine has been smoked or chewed in various preparations of tobacco, both for ceremonial purposes and for producing altered states of consciousness. Addictive patterns of compulsive use have also been reported for centuries. The history of nicotine use indicates various applications in daily life and even in medicine. The history of the tobacco trade is rich and has many parallels with the opium wars of the 19th century and with the illicit cocaine trade of the 20th century. The history of nicotine use also demonstrates important behavioral and psychosocial influences on tobacco use and its spread. The history of attempts to remove tobacco from various societies provides a basis for attempting to formulate policy in today's world.

Chapter 3: Who Smokes and What Kills Them

Tobacco use caused approximately 3 million deaths per year worldwide in the 1990s and could result in approximately 1 billion premature deaths between 1900 and 2100. The spread of tobacco use resembles the diffusion of other "innovations." Tobacco use is becoming concentrated in certain populations in the United States, such as less educated white persons. Unfortunately, few societies have been as effective at curbing the spread of tobacco use as they have been at curbing diseases mediated by bacteria and viruses. In part, this is because of the dependence-producing drug nicotine, which alters the behavior of tobacco users such that the users themselves resist disease eradication efforts. Death rates tell just part of the story. Most people who smoke are sick more often, using about two more sick days per year than do nonsmokers. Many people who die prematurely because of tobacco get sick first and require years or months of costly treatment. Heart disease kills more smokers than any other smoking-related disease. The risk of contracting heart disease is most effectively reduced by quitting smoking.

Trends and projections regarding tobacco use and disease along with the behavioral epidemiology of tobacco dependence are discussed from a worldwide perspective, with an emphasis on the United States.

Chapter 4: What Nicotine Does to the Body

People may start smoking to achieve certain images and social status, but soon the effects of nicotine on the body become an important part of the experience. Nicotine is a potent and powerful drug with many effects. Nicotine is about 10 times more potent, milligram for milligram, than cocaine or morphine. Nicotine is *psychoactive* (or psychologically active) and affects behavior; in high doses, it is deadly, which is why it is used as an insecticide.

Portions of the human nervous system were mapped using nicotine as a type of chemical tracer early in the 20th century. A fuller understanding of the diverse actions of nicotine in the brain came only after the development of various neuropharmacological techniques during the latter half of the 20th century. This research has revealed that nicotine produces a cascade of effects, including causing the body to develop extra nicotine receptors, activating some of the same neurotransmitter systems as are activated by cocaine, modulating cerebral metabolic activity in the brain, and altering the brain's electrophysiological activity. This research has revealed many of the underlying effects on the brain, the nervous system, and the endocrine system. All of those effects contribute to the observed behavioral effects of nicotine, including addiction. Understanding some of the basic chemistry underlying the effects of nicotine is not only fascinating but provides a foundation for material covered in the remainder of the book.

Chapter 5: The Natural History of a Dependence Disorder

Biological and psychosocial influences conspire to determine the natural history of cigarette smoking. Cigarettes provide opportunities for social interaction, and nicotine stimulates reward pathways in the brain, but these aspects of smoking provide only part of the story of why people smoke. People can obtain a wide variety of what they perceive as useful effects from nicotine, which can add to the difficulty they may experience in quitting smoking and sustaining abstinence. Extensive research on the behavioral pharmacology of nicotine in nonhuman animals and in humans has revealed that nicotine can readily modify behavior through a variety of mechanisms. For example, nicotine exposure can directly enhance the rate of certain ongoing behaviors while disrupting the rate of other behaviors. Its administration can elicit a variety of responses, ranging from nausea to pleasant mood states. The rich array of behavioral effects provided by nicotine enables the drug to modulate a wide range of behaviors, including powerful drug-seeking behavior. The size of a nicotine dose is an important determinant of the effects of nicotine.

Chapter 6: Tobacco Use as Nicotine Addiction

Nicotine exposure can lead to tolerance, physical dependence, and compulsive use, even when the user knows that tobacco is harmful. The clinical characteristics of nicotine dependence are discussed within the broader conceptual framework of drug dependence as a behavioral disorder, as well as from the medical perspective of drug-use diagnosis. The history of the terms *addiction* and *dependence* are examined. This section also compares the dependence properties of nicotine with those of other addicting drugs, such as opioids (e.g., heroin) and cocaine.

Chapter 7: Smoking, Drinking, and Drug Taking: A Biobehavioral Syndrome

The puzzling syndromes of multiple drug use and risky behavior patterns are explored in this chapter. We discuss the involvement of smoking in other behavioral disorders, with special emphasis on what is known about the causative role of tobacco use in other behaviors.

Chapter 8: "Low-Tar," "Light" Cigarettes: Lessons From a Dangerous Boondoggle

The cigarette is an extremely sophisticated drug delivery system that can easily support addiction in smokers. Because of a flawed and inaccurate testing and labeling system, some cigarettes are labeled "low-tar" or "light." These light and low-tar cigarettes have been marketed to retain health-conscious smokers among the ranks of smokers. This chapter explains why the risks of smoking are not substantially reduced by the introduction of low-yield cigarettes. This chapter also provides an opportunity to explain the cigarette as a drug delivery system. Cigarette engineering and smoking behavior are presented in detail in this chapter.

Chapter 9: Helping Smokers Quit

Many treatment strategies have evolved over the past three decades, from intuitive approaches practiced more as art than medicine to rationally based strategies with more predictable outcomes. Understanding what works and what doesn't work in helping people quit smoking provides further insights about the nature of the dependence disorder. This chapter explains how nicotine dependence can be treated using individual behavioral interventions and medications. Research on what are called *brief interventions* in primary care settings, such as doctors' and dentists' offices, is also explored.

Chapter 10: Smoking, Public Health, and Policy

The preceding chapters have provided the foundation for discussions about future policy options. At the societal level, how can we prevent people from starting smoking, and how can we help smokers quit? This chapter presents a variety of strategies. The importance of having both effective and practical strategies will be emphasized. Unfortunately, some of the schemes (for example, low-tar cigarettes) for reducing the health costs of smoking have, in contrast, been counterproductive.

Summary

A biobehavioral approach is fundamentally interdisciplinary or multidisciplinary, even transdisciplinary. Also, biological and behavioral domains are distinct. In addition, a biobehavioral approach values research studies that include consideration of both biological and behavioral influences. Cigarette smoking is the largest preventable cause of death and disability in many developed countries and is a dramatically growing problem in less-developed countries of the world. Nicotine is the key ingredient in all popular forms of tobacco (cigarettes, smokeless tobacco, cigars and pipes) and is largely responsible for the continued use of tobacco in spite of the costs to health. This book reviews the research literature on nicotine and health, with an emphasis on cigarettes because of their widespread use and adverse health effects. The major health consequences of smoking arise out of the interplay of cigarettes and nicotine.

Further Reading

Kozlowski, L. T., & Herman, C. P. (1984). The interaction of psychosocial and biological determinants of tobacco use: More on the boundary model. *Journal of Applied Social Psychology, 14,* 244-256.

This article gives an example of the importance of jointly considering psychosocial (behavioral) and biological determinants of smoking.

U.S. Department of Health, Education, and Welfare. (1979). *Smoking and health: A report of the surgeon general* (DHEW Publication No. PHS 79-50066). Washington, DC: U.S. Department of Health, Education, and Welfare, Public Health Service, Office of the Assistant Secretary for Health, Office on Smoking and Health.

This landmark report was released 15 years after the first surgeon general's report in 1964. The 1979 report is the largest of the surgeon general's reports and includes many excellent review chapters on both biological and behavioral factors related to cigarette smoking.

2

The History of the Use of Nicotine

A Tasty Wonder Drug
for Many, if Not All, Occasions

Gods would have revell'd at their feats of Mirth
With this pure distillation of the Earth;
The Marrow of the World, Star of the West,
The Pearl whereby this lower Orb is blest;
The Joy of Mortals, Umpire of all Strife,
Delight of Nature, Mithradate[1] of Life;
The daintiest dish of a delicious feast,
By taking which Man differs from a beast.

"The Smoky Magic"
Anonymous (poem from early 1600s)
(Partington, 1925, p. 159)

When cured in the right way, a leaf of tobacco looks like gold. It folds like money, and a deep, sweet, rich smell rises from it. Much of tobacco's history has been written by loving fans of this "golden leaf." Some of the early authors—without the scientific knowledge of the diseases caused by tobacco use and without any need to give up tobacco—may not have been aware that drug taking and drug addiction were central elements of their devotion to the product. Several interesting books, each several times the length of this book, document tobacco's major influence on culture, literature, art, and the economy (see Further Reading at the end of this chapter).

It can be easy to dismiss historical perspectives by adopting the notion "that was then, this is now." The history presented here will show that much of the "now" is remarkably like the "then." In the United States, tobacco is used by a sizable minority of the adult population. However, tobacco is also stigmatized and is not nearly as socially acceptable as it was 30 or 40 years ago. This suggests that, for the majority of the readers of this book, smoking is a minor issue, of direct interest only to other people. But consider that tobacco use—wherever it has been introduced—has become a core part of a society's cultural and economic life. Tobacco has been used literally as currency in some cultures, and tobacco use has thrived even in cultures where people lost their heads to the executioner's blade if caught smoking. *A plant that not only kills people (see Chapter 3), but that many people also have died for, demands attention.*

The birthplace of tobacco as a cultivated plant is the Americas. The best evidence about early, preindustrial uses of tobacco comes from studies of native peoples of North and South America. Three basic themes, the first two biological and the third behavioral, emerge:

1. All popular tobacco products have been drug delivery devices for nicotine.
2. As do popular foods and drinks, most popular tobacco products have pleasing tastes and smells.
3. Cultural, situational, and psychosocial factors strongly influence how various societies have viewed and used tobacco products.

Several different types of tobacco products have been popular during the last 500 years. Each of these products, except for the modern cigarette, has a long history of use.

Nicotine becomes available through the harvesting and processing of tobacco leaves. Just as there are varieties of apples, there are varieties of tobacco. The plant kingdom is divided into families, which are then divided into *genera* and further subdivided into *species*. *Nicotiana* plants are members of a family of plants called the Solanaceae, also called nightshades. The nightshades include other poisonous plants (tobacco is poisonous), such as the deadly nightshade, as well as food plants such as potatoes, tomatoes, and peppers. Among the genus of *nicotiana* are dozens of species. By far, the two most important species are *nicotiana rustica* and *nicotiana tabacum*. *Rustica* can be likened to a harsh, sour apple that needs to be cooked and sweetened before eating, and *tabacum* can be likened to a mild, sweet variety of apple that is edible when picked from the tree. *Rustica* is the rawer, less palatable form of tobacco; *tabacum* has greater consumer acceptability. Figure 2.1 shows the first published illustration of *nicotiana tabacum*. These tobacco plants are native to the Americas and have been spread around the world by persons interested in using or selling processed tobacco.

The difference between these two species of tobacco plants—*rustica* versus *tabacum*—played a key role in the commercial history of tobacco. Tobacco exported from the Spanish colonies in the New World was *tabacum* rather than *rustica*. Tobacco from the British colonies was at first the less prized *rustica*. The importation by John Rolfe of *nicotiana tabacum* seeds to the Jamestown Colony in Virginia in 1613 allowed the British colonies to grow and market *tabacum* (Herndon, 1957). They thereby became much more competitive in the tobacco business. The modern commercial tobacco crop in the southern United States is based on the growing of *nicotiana tabacum*.

Types of Tobacco Products

Smokeless Tobacco Products

Unsmoked tobacco products have been popular in three types: chewing tobacco, wet snuff, and dry snuff. *Chewing tobacco* (also, chew or chaw) is used either in a plug or in loose form. The plug is a compressed, flavored bar of processed tobacco; other chewing tobacco is usually flavored, coarsely chopped tobacco. These products are put in the mouth and chewed. *Wet snuff* (also, *moist snuff, dipping tobacco,* or *dip*) is also put in the mouth, but it is finely chopped, moist, and flavored and is placed between the cheek and gums, where the nicotine is ab-

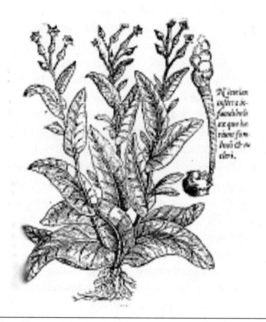

Figure 2.1. First Published Illustration of *Nicotiana Tabacum*
SOURCE: Pena and l'Obel (1571). Image published with permission of Bell & Howell Information and Learning Company. Further reproduction is prohibited without permission.
NOTE: The small head and tube of tobacco leaves on the right is described (in Latin) as indicating how tobacco is used by Indians and sailors.

sorbed through the lining of the mouth. Sometimes brushes made of chewed twigs are used to apply the moist tobacco to the mouth. Oral smokeless tobacco products are also called "spit tobacco," because they stimulate saliva production and lead to spitting. *Dry snuff* (also, *sniffing snuff*) is a very fine, dry, scented powder of tobacco with a consistency similar to ground cinnamon. Dry snuff is snorted or snuffed into the nose, where nicotine is absorbed from the lining of the nasal passages into the bloodstream. See Chapter 4 for more on pharmacokinetics (the movement of drugs through the body and brain).

Pipes and Cigars

Pipe tobacco is finely chopped tobacco that often has been scented or flavored. Clay or carved stone pipes have been found in ancient archaeological sites.

Cigars are the wrapped leaves of specially cured tobacco. Adequate doses of nicotine are usually gotten through the oral tissues without having to inhale the smoke. Inhalation refers to taking tobacco smoke into the lungs.

Cigarettes

The modern cigarette was developed in the late 1800s, using the so-called bright or flue-cured tobacco leaf, which produced a product that was easy to inhale. Inhaled smoke is an extremely effective way to get nicotine into the bloodstream and quickly into the brain.

■ Drug Delivery Devices

All popular forms of tobacco are ways for people to use the drug nicotine. No form of tobacco use that fails to deliver doses of nicotine to the brain has been popular. Though the forms of tobacco (e.g., chewing tobacco, wet snuff, dry snuff, tobacco, pipe, cigars, or cigarettes) differ in the route efficiency and speed of getting nicotine to the brain, they all can do the job as they are typically used.

A drug that affects the brain is called a *psychoactive* drug. Although modern research has demonstrated the psychoactivity of nicotine, anyone who has ever tried a tobacco product and felt lightheaded or dizzy has experienced firsthand the psychoactivity of nicotine. Nicotine's action as a stimulant has no doubt contributed to its popularity. The earliest European accounts describe tobacco being used by the native people to fight fatigue and hunger. Today, nicotine is used as a stimulant by many truck drivers, by students studying late before a test, or by others wanting to feel alert and awake.

■ Popular Forms of Tobacco
Taste and Smell Good to Users

For the most part, tobacco is not just grown, cut, dried, and sold to the consumer. It is processed, cured, and "cooked," in much the same way that foods are prepared. Just as a chocolate bar is not simply raw chocolate, popular tobacco products are not raw tobacco. Tobacco products, to be effective drug delivery devices, are manufactured to be pleasant tasting and pleasant smelling. Sauces, flavorings, honey, and sugars are among the ingredients in popular tobacco products. The sailors traveling with Columbus, observing native people smoking, noted that the "Indian" had with him dry leaves which "they esteem for their *odor* [italics added] and healthfulness" (quoted in Dickson, 1954, p. 102). The first recorded accounts of tobacco preparation described detailed procedures for curing and flavoring tobacco products. In the early days of cigarette advertising, slogans often invoked issues of flavorings and tastes (see Lewine, 1970):

"A dash of chocolate."
"Your nose knows."
"You can make yourself the mildest, most fragrant cigarette in the world."
"Reach for a Lucky instead of a sweet."
"It's toasted."
"Smoke Omar for Aroma."
"45 minutes toasting develops its aristocratic flavor."

Today, the most popular cigarette tobaccos are subjected to a high-temperature "toasting" process that enhances the natural sugar content of tobacco. The most popular cigarette in the world, Marlboro, is a complex blend of different tobaccos and flavoring sauces.

Taste and smell are known as the chemical senses. These senses connect to noncognitive parts of the human brain also common in other animals and have strong effects on behavior. Bad-tasting, bad-smelling foods are shunned by all but the hungriest persons. A delicious food (e.g., a dessert at the end of a meal) can tempt further eating in someone who is full. Stimulation of the chemical senses adds to the pleasures of tobacco use, and it encourages and enables the tobacco user to control the intake of the drugs in tobacco. Someone who self-administers an unknown drug by injection with a syringe has few cues to help determine the correct dose. On the other hand, each cigarette puff produces strong sensations that the smoker uses to estimate and control the amount of tobacco and nicotine being consumed. A great deal of research on drug taking shows that users prefer to be able to predict and control the doses of the drugs they take. The tastes and smells of most popular forms of tobacco allow such prediction and control.

The chemical senses are responsible for triggering so-called *cephalic phase responses* in the body (Powley, 1977). (*Cephalic* refers to the head.) When substances are tasted, they can produce strong biological reactions that prepare the body for processing foods. Likewise, tobacco in the mouth or nose can stimulate cephalic phase responses that may contribute to the way the body reacts to the tobacco.

The varied tastes and smells of tobacco products also provide a basis for personal preferences and connoisseurship. The quest for the most pleasing, best-tasting product has been part of the history of tobacco (in this it can be compared to the culture of fine wines). Much of the literature of tobacco use celebrates the tastes and smells of prepared tobaccos (e.g., Bain, 1896; Elwa, 1974; Partington, 1925).

◼ Early Indications of Addiction

Even the earliest accounts of tobacco use suggest that nicotine is dependence producing, or addictive. *A central feature of an addiction is difficulty in going without the use of the product* (Kalant, Clarke, Corrigall, Ferrence, & Kozlowski, 1989). The first European observations of tobacco use were made in 1492 by two sailors in the crew of Christopher Columbus. The sailors noticed that many local people constantly carried a "burning torch" to set fire to certain herbs (tobacco) that they carried with them (Dickson, 1954, p. 105). In 1586, an early French traveler to Brazil, Jean De Léry, described a kind of cigar smoking by the native people. He noted that tobacco was greatly valued by them and added, "You will never see the Brazilians when they do not each have a tube of this plant hanging around their necks" (cited in Dickson, 1954, p. 128). De Léry also explained that they kept puffing on tubes of tobacco even while conversing.

In what is now Canada, at roughly the same time, French explorer Jacques Cartier (1545), offered a similar account of the local smoking customs:

> They also have a plant of *which they gather a great supply in the summer to last during the winter.* This they *prize very much,* and only men use it, in the following manner. They dry it in the sun and carry it on their necks in a small animal skin, instead of a bag, with a pipe of stone or wood. Then *frequently* they make a powder of this plant, putting it on one of the ends of the pipe and laying a coal of fire on it they suck at the other end until they fill their bodies with smoke, so that it come out of their mouths and nostrils like a chimney. And *they say that this keeps them healthy and warm and they never go anywhere without these things* [italics added throughout]. (quoted in Dickson, 1954, p. 116)

Cartier was writing an account for readers who had never seen pipes or pipe smoking.

The first clear description of addiction to tobacco by Europeans is that of Las Casas in the 1500s. Just a few decades after Columbus arrived in America, during

the colonization of Haiti (Hispaniola), Las Casas saw Spaniards who used tobacco and who "were not able to stop taking" tobacco, in spite of tobacco use being called a vice and in spite of the Spaniards' being criticized for not stopping
(Dickson, 1954, p. 105).

■ Cultural, Situational, and Psychosocial Factors

An anthropologist (Ortiz, 1947) once argued that pipes suited sedentary societies,
cigars suited ambulatory societies, and cigarettes were most at home in impatient
societies. Consider this claim. Pipes are easiest to smoke when one is sitting and
when one has easy access to sources of fire, because pipes often need to be relit.
Bouncing along on horseback is not a suitable setting for smoking a pipe. However, a cigar smoker can light a cigar and go for a long walk, because a long cigar
might take 30 to 45 minutes to smoke, hardly something to squeeze into a 10-min-
ute wait for a bus. Requiring only about 8 minutes to smoke, a cigarette provides a
quick hit of nicotine.

What is or is not convenient differs from society to society and from time to
time. The invention of the match or the portable lighter, the enactment of local
laws against smoking in restaurants, and the supply of free cigarettes to soldiers
during wartime have profoundly changed the convenience of various tobacco
products.

■ Early Use of Tobacco in the Americas

Early tobacco use can be divided into three categories: (a) ritual or spiritual, (b)
medicinal, and (c) everyday or recreational.

Ritual or Spiritual Tobacco Use

Myths about the origins of tobacco abound. Tobacco was not a side issue
but was the fundamental plant used in dealings with the supernatural by the Native
Americans from North America to the tip of South America (La Barre, 1972).
Though tobacco was often seen as a gift from supernatural beings (e.g., Great
Spirit, Manitous, the Earthmaker, or the Creator), it was viewed as more than a

simple present from the gods. Rather, it was a gift that created an ongoing connection and relationship between people and the gods. Tobacco provided a way for human beings to please supernatural powers. A common belief in the Americas was that the Creator or the Spirits had a special love for tobacco, but they could not grow tobacco themselves. They needed humans to provide them with tobacco. In return for producing smoke for these supernatural beings, the human beings would be fed and protected (Callender, 1978; Tooker, 1979; Wilbert, 1987).

In some formulations, tobacco was seen explicitly as the food of the gods—the only thing that the Manitous ate, a food for which the gods felt a strong hunger or craving (Wilbert, 1987). Tobacco thus facilitated a sacred interdependence between humans and their spirit world. Human beings needed the Spirits to provide food and water for them; the Spirits were tobacco lovers (addicts) dependent on human beings to be their drug suppliers. These beliefs about the desires and cravings of the gods may have arisen from the direct human experience of the pleasures and effects of nicotine and from the reactions of the devoted human user of tobacco to periods of separation from tobacco.

Within such a belief system, tobacco was a crucial commodity. Giving tobacco to the Spirits could be seen as a core ritual for the community—a ritual necessary for the maintenance of human life in a dangerous world.

Some tobacco myths from South America pointed to a distinction between "good" tobacco and "bad" tobacco (Lévi-Strauss, 1973). Bad tobacco was tobacco seen as a deadly poison that could transform humans into undesirable animals (e.g., anteaters). Good tobacco could transform a shaman or priest into a jaguar—a powerful, magical, treasured animal. Shamans used tobacco as a strong, dangerous drug. High doses of nicotine caused trances, stupors, loss of consciousness, convulsions, hallucinations, and visions (Wilbert, 1987). During these intoxicated states, the shamans communicated with the gods and received visions that guided their later actions. Training as a shaman often would involve repeated exposure to ever-increasing doses of tobacco. The large, intoxicating doses of tobacco that were consumed could have killed (and must have sometimes killed) these shamanic users. In other words, by employing strong doses of tobacco, shamans were using poison to skirt the deadly edges of life and consciousness.

Many tribes intentionally grew tobacco rather than depending on finding it in the wild. Even tribes that did not grow other plants or crops were likely to grow tobacco. The growing of tobacco was sometimes seen as a privilege, the job of the males. In some groups, only males were permitted to use tobacco.

Tobacco as Medicine

Perhaps because it sounds so different from prevailing contemporary uses of tobacco, the ritual uses of tobacco by indigenous peoples of the Americas intrigue us. The medicinal uses were related to the ritual holy uses; the tobacco visions of the shaman were often a search for a cure for illness or affliction. Tobacco was used to fight hunger and fatigue. Tobacco was also widely used to treat disease and wounds. Often, the shaman would blow smoke on the afflicted person as part of a ritual healing process.

Modern science has clarified that tobacco is certainly not a cure-all. Some of tobacco's apparent effects on disease may have been due to a *placebo effect,* such that with belief in the medicine, an ineffective substance can contribute to cures. Because nicotine was producing strong physiological responses, it was an *active placebo* that did have perceptible effects on the body and mind.

In addition, a discussion of ritual and medicinal uses of tobacco can easily obscure the fact that tobacco was probably widely used on a daily basis by many native persons. The great abundance of clay pipes at native archaeological sites suggests that pipe smoking was hardly reserved only for the shaman or used only on special occasions (von Gernet, 2000).

■ Tobacco in Europe

Imagine what it was like to have been among the first small group in your hometown to have tobacco or to know how to use tobacco. Erase any modern negative images you have of tobacco. When it was first introduced in Europe, tobacco was seen as a wonder drug that took away hunger and fatigue and cured diseases. Sailors, the world travelers of the 1500s, spread tobacco as a kind of "street drug" they tried in the Americas and brought home to Europe as a prized novelty. The fad spread from port to port in a classic pattern by which new products or innovations are often diffused across the world (compare Rogers, 1983).

By the mid-1500s, tobacco was creating great interest not only as a medicine but as a panacea that could cure ailments and sores that physicians had declared incurable. It was noticed by Jean Nicot, a French ambassador to Portugal. At the time Nicot discovered tobacco, Portugal was a leading world power with a major merchant navy and colonies (e.g., Brazil) in South America. Nicot knew that herbalists were growing tobacco and that pharmacists were selling tobacco leaves as medicine. He praised the curative powers of tobacco as he spoke to key members of the clergy and court in France. He sent tobacco seeds and plants to France. Solutions of tobacco were used to treat asthma and assorted skin ailments. Nicotine, the primary pharmacological agent in tobacco, was named after Nicot.

Spain was also one the most powerful nations in Europe at this time. In the 1570s, Nicolás Monardés, an influential Spanish physician, published an authoritative book on medicines from the West Indies. Tobacco was touted as an amazing cure-all. At great length, Monardés explained the use of tobacco products to treat nearly every know human malady. It was recommended as a remedy for thirst, hunger, weakness, worms, asthma, stomach ailments, toothaches, sores, respiratory illness, painful joints, headaches, wounds, bleeding, stiff neck, and even bad breath. Monardés's book was much cited by advocates for tobacco use, and for about 100 years it was considered the definitive medical statement on tobacco's virtues.

Tobacco in England

Tobacco came to England in the 1560s and 1570s. In 1577, Monardés's book was translated into English. At a higher social level, tobacco was presented at the Royal Court and circulated among the aristocracy by early explorers and importers, including Sir Walter Raleigh. According to a story, Raleigh, one of the first smokers in England, was thought to be on fire when smoking, and a servant threw water on him to put the fire out. At a lower social level, sailors again were instrumental in the introduction of tobacco to England.

Within just 30 years, tobacco use grew dramatically, and cultivation of tobacco in England became common. Tobacco use became fashionable and trendy. Historians and poets praised tobacco. But by 1600, a backlash against tobacco was starting. No less than the king of England attempted to counteract the popularity of tobacco. King James I, also responsible for commissioning the King James Version of the Christian Bible, proposed a heavy tax of 4,000% on tobacco. The king defended this tax by arguing that, while the right sort of people were not misusing tobacco, a growing number of persons were suffering the ruin of their estates to keep themselves supplied with tobacco. The tax was intended to discourage self-abusive tobacco use and may have been the first tax law created to control drug use in a population.

King James I (1604/1954) wrote the single most famous essay in English against tobacco use, *The Counter-Blaste Against Tobacco*. The prominence of tobacco as a growing fashion in England must have been substantial to warrant the personal attention of the king. The most quoted passage from the *Counter-Blaste* is the conclusion, which condemns tobacco smoking as "A custome loathsome to the eye, hateful to the Nose, harmefull to the braine, dangerous to the Lungs, and the blacke stinking fume thereof, neerest resembling the horrible Stigian smoke of the pit that is bottomlesse" (p. 36). This comparison of tobacco smoke with the smoke of hell resembles the more modern tactics of arguing that tobacco smoke is unhealthful and even sinful.

A close look at the entire essay shows that the king was upset at the popularity of this alien-born fashion. He was upset that his people were emulating Indians (some of whom were slaves of the Spanish), the French, and the Spanish. He argued that the medical claims for tobacco were unproven, noting that sick people often got well on their own and that it would be illogical to attribute all cures to the effects of tobacco. Most interesting to us is the emphasis that King James I placed on tobacco as a dependence-producing substance. He described heavy users as becoming tolerant to the effects of tobacco, referring to this reduced effect from tobacco as a "bewitching" quality. He said that smokers related to tobacco as drunkards related to alcohol; users were said to have a "sinneful and shameful lust" for tobacco.

The king offered a view of the sin of drunkenness in keeping with modern knowledge of dependence on psychoactive drugs: "Tobacco abuse is a branche of the sinne of drunkeness, which is the roote of all sinnes: for as the onely delight that drunkards take in wine is in the strength of the taste, and the force of the fume thereof that mounts up to the brain" (p. 29). Another passage also captures the opinion that tobacco is an addictive substance that users have trouble going without: "Many in this kingdome have had such continual use of taking this unsavorie smoke, as now they are unable to forbeare the same, no more than an old drunkard can abide to be sober, without falling into an uncurable weakenesse and evill constitution" (p. 27). King James I also notes that this acquired "habit" becomes second nature to users.

As remarkable as the king's opposition to tobacco was the king's dramatic change in policy toward tobacco. After just a few years, the king may have realized that tobacco use was unstoppable, that a more reasonable tax would bring money into the royal treasury, and that the Virginia colony needed tobacco exports. Whatever the mixture of reasons, the strong royal objection to tobacco was abandoned, and tobacco became an important moneymaker for the government. This pattern of initial resistance followed by official acceptance became a pattern that occurred throughout Europe and much of the rest of the world.

A Pattern of Growth, Rejection, and Acceptance

Studies of the introduction of tobacco into Italy, France, Turkey, Russia, Japan, and China in the 1600s reveal remarkably consistent patterns. First, tobacco popularity grew rapidly. Tobacco was everywhere promoted as a wonder drug, a precious herb that could cure otherwise incurable diseases. Clearly, its properties as a stimulant were prized. Tobacco use became fashionable and was adopted by individuals interested in following current fashions. Cultivation was widespread.

Typically, authorities then tried to end or reduce tobacco use. Tobacco was viewed as an evil foreign product corrupting citizens and jeopardizing a country's welfare. The response in England was fairly tame compared with that in the rest of the world. In Italy, the Pope ruled that users of tobacco would be excommunicated (thrown out of the Catholic Church) for using tobacco. The clergy themselves in Spain and Italy used tobacco during sacred rituals (e.g., the mass) despite orders not to smoke or chew tobacco in the church. (These rules had loopholes that kept them from being taken seriously.) In Turkey, the rulers placed a stiff penalty on tobacco use: A pipe stem was forced through the nose of the tobacco user, and the offender was paraded through the streets to display this disfigurement. A later Turkish ruler (Murad IV, the Cruel, 1623-1640) blamed a major fire on tobacco users and ordered that all tobacco taverns be destroyed and all users be killed. Many smokers were beheaded, their estates enriching the royal treasury. In Russia, smokers were whipped or their noses were slit with a knife; repeat offenders were sent penniless into exile in Siberia. Prison terms and property confiscation were penalties in Japan for the use of tobacco. In China, convicted tobacco dealers were beheaded. In the face of growing drug abuse, societies throughout history have exacted extreme punishments for drug use (e.g., in our day, life sentences without possibility of parole for drug dealing). In no case has dire punishment put an end to the drug abuse, and in every situation cited here, tobacco use continued to spread.

As a final step in this pattern, severe restrictions were abandoned. Tobacco was transformed into a legal product with few restrictions on its use. The practice became further entrenched in various societies. For example, in early colonial society in North America, tobacco was legal tender and could be used to pay any lawful debt (Young, 1916). Governments made money from tobacco taxes and government monopolies on the sale of tobacco (Austin, 1978). The foreign crop became a domestic product. Even so, societal acceptance of tobacco was not unflagging, and tobacco prohibition movements grew. The most famous physician in the United States, Dr. Benjamin Rush of Philadelphia (a signer of the Declaration of Independence) wrote the first substantial antitobacco work in the country in 1798. One of his main concerns was the powerful link between tobacco abuse and alcohol abuse. Religious and medical professionals spoke out against tobacco use. In the mid 1880s, a British medical journal, *The Lancet,* carried an influential series of letters debating the pros and cons of tobacco use.

Chewing tobacco was a convenient form of tobacco use for a largely rural culture that often demanded two-handed work in flammable environments. The public streets of the time were ripe with the smell and debris of horse manure (but no auto emissions), and the sidewalks were stained with the tobacco juice and spit-out wads (quids) of tobacco. Though many commentators saw this widespread public expectoration (spitting) as vile and disgusting, the disapproval had little effect on the practice. Spitting of tobacco was reported in churches, streetcars, railway cars, and courthouses. Contemporary accounts noted that the long skirts of women were often soiled by being dragged through the juicy mounds of tobacco on the floors in public places. Women's distaste for the detritus of spit tobacco was a force behind some antitobacco prohibitions, such as a condemnation of tobacco in the early Mormon Church in 1833. It was not until the late 19th century that the theory of germs was developed, and scientists and health professionals realized that public spitting was spreading disease. Antispitting laws were passed in New York and Philadelphia in 1896. Concern about the unhygienic practice of public spitting undoubtedly reduced the convenience of chewing tobacco. Along with the rise of the modern cigarette, these health concerns promoted a decline of the use of chewing tobacco in the United States.

■ The Modern Cigarette

One of the most famous names in the history of the modern cigarette is James Bonsack, the inventor of an effective machine for mass-producing cigarettes. In 1883, James Buchanan ("Buck") Duke started using this machine to make cigarettes. Within a year, the machine was making 120,000 cigarettes a day, compared with a little over 2,000 a day that could be done by those who rolled cigarettes by hand. The manufactured cigarette expanded the reach of cigarette manufacturers. Buck Duke is believed to have originated the idea for picture cards of celebrities (actresses, baseball players, or other athletes) being added to cigarette packages as a promotional device. The most valuable, collectable "baseball card" did not come with bubble gum but cigarettes, and it became rare because the star, Honus Wagner, insisted his picture not be so used, because he was against smoking.

In the late 1890s, Lucy Page Gaston started the influential Anti-Cigarette League. This group helped pass total antismoking bans in several state legislatures. At one point, about one fourth of all states, particularly those in the Midwest, totally banned smoking. Even more states had bans on the sale of cigarettes to young people. Celebrities endorsed abstinence from cigarettes. Some historians estimate that these anticigarette efforts did cause a temporary decline in cigarette use (Brooks, 1953). As a foreshadowing of the present polarized public positions about tobacco, one anonymous tobacco executive stated in 1916:

> No intelligent manufacturer objects to the enactment and enforcement of state laws prohibiting the sale of cigarettes to minors. We do not. In fact we heartily encourage such legislation.
>
> Naturally we object to sweeping prohibitive laws that deny grown men the right to smoke what they please. (Young, 1916, p. 271)

Comparing the current tobacco debates with those of more than a half-century ago, we see a repeated pattern of battle between pro- and antitobacco interests, creating an oscillation in societal encouragement and discouragement of tobacco use. The current antismoking movement benefits from the weight of sound scientific evidence that, in retrospect, prior restrictive movements lacked. But the oscillating pattern may not end with scientific debate in developed countries, because protobacco forces remain dominant in many developing countries around the world. Ironically, it is as if tobacco use is both an important problem that must be stopped and an important advantage that cannot be stopped: Widespread smoking is expensive to encourage, but its profits are too much too lose. This situation is reminiscent of the old joke about John, who had a brother, Ned, who thought he was a chicken. When John was discussing the problem with a psychiatrist, the psychiatrist said that Ned should be hospitalized. John said he was not willing to hospitalize his brother, because he had grown dependent on the eggs. Though one

TABLE 2.1 Some Historic Variations On and One Prediction About Popular Nicotine Use Practices

Time Period	Region	Tobacco Product	Preferred Mode of Use
1. 1600s	United Kingdom	Pipe	Smoke in mouth
2. 1700s	Most of Europe	Dry snuff	Tobacco up nose
3. 1800s	North America	Chewing tobacco	Tobacco in mouth
4. 1900s	The world	Cigarettes	Smoke in lungs
5. 2000s	The world	Cigarettes or alternative nicotine delivery systems	Smoke in lungs or nicotine vapor in nose or lungs

part of our society wants to eliminate tobacco in society, another part of society cannot afford to be without the money from tobacco.

The Rise of Advertising

In the United States in 1912, the first national advertising campaign was launched for a cigarette (Camel). Shortly thereafter, national ad campaigns promoted Lucky Strike and Chesterfield. These three brands dominated cigarette sales for the next 50 years. Lucky Strike packages proclaimed, "It's toasted." Before this time, cigarette advertising was limited to local promotion of regional brands. In the second decade of the 20th century, World War I also contributed to the dramatic growth in smoking and the popularity of the cigarette. At one point in World War I, the United States government bought an entire production of Bull Durham tobacco and sent the tobacco and cigarette paper to the U.S. troops. The shipments bore written slogans: "When our boys light up, the Huns will light out" (i.e., the Germans will run away) and "The Makings for US, The Leavings for the Kaiser!"

Summary

Tobacco has been used in varied ways over the last 400 years (see Table 2.1). The variations show how culture can influence the form of tobacco use. When Americans in the United States were chewing tobacco and spitting wherever they pleased, the British and the French were stuffing powdered tobacco up their noses. Contemporary histories indicate that users were attached to their particular manner of use and were contemptuous of other ways of using tobacco. Whereas one writer would describe chewing tobacco as delicious, another who was sniffing tobacco would describe chewing tobacco as revolting (Kozlowski, 1982). The last row of Table 2.1 raises the issue of the future of alternative nicotine delivery systems (see Chapter 10 for more on this), but acknowledges that cigarettes will still likely be around. Tobacco products (nicotine delivery systems) in all their variety have had a long and resilient history. They could be with us, in some form, long into the future.

▓ Note

1. Mithradate is an antidote for poison.

Further Reading

Austin, G. A. (1978). *Perspectives on the history of psychoactive substance use.* Rockville, MD: National Institute on Drug Abuse.

This is an excellent overview of the history of psychoactive substances around the world.

Goodman, J. (1993). *Tobacco in history: The cultures of dependence.* London: Routledge.

This is a more recent world history of tobacco use.

Robert, J. C. (1949). *The story of tobacco in America.* Chapel Hill: University of North Carolina Press.

This is an entertaining, scholarly history of tobacco use in the United States.

Wilbert, J. (1987). *Tobacco and Shamanism in South America.* New Haven, CT: Yale University Press.

This anthropological work describes the use of tobacco by native peoples in South America.

Winter, J. C. (Ed.) (2001). *Tobacco use by native North Americans: Sacred smoke and silent killer.* Norman, OK: University of Oklahoma Press.

3

Who Smokes and What Kills Them

Women who smoke like men die like men who smoke.

> —U.S. Department of Health,
> Education, and Welfare (1979)

This chapter is about life and death—the product life of cigarettes and the early death of persons. Cigarettes have had different lives in different countries. In the United States in the 20th century, the modern cigarette flourished once, then dwindled, but began to show signs of new growth among the young at the close of the century. Smoking came into fashion first for men, then for women, and fell out of fashion, first for men, then for women (Ferrence, 1990). Social pressures brought individuals to smoking and then, similar, but opposing, social pressures pushed people away from smoking. We will trace the dynamic career of the modern cigarette through the 20th century with an emphasis on the United States but also with attention to what happened elsewhere in the world.

The fatality rates of smokers have followed the rises and falls in popularity of cigarettes with a delay in time. This delay arises (a) out of the decades it can take for cigarettes to cause disease (heart disease, lung cancer, emphysema, bronchitis, other cancers) and (b) the further years it takes for those diseases to kill smokers. The public health costs of a product are a function of both the health risks of using a product as it is typically used and the number of users of the product. Epidemiology is the study of the spread of human disease through time (past, present, and projected into the future) and space (e.g., males vs. females, groups, countries). Behavioral epidemiology concerns the spread of behaviors (e.g., cigarette smoking) that cause human disease. If only 1% of adults had used cigarettes from the 1920s to the 1960s in the United States or if most of those who smoked did so only now and then, the body count from smoking-caused disease would not justify this book. The historic reports of the Royal College of Physicians in Britain or of the surgeons general of the United States would not have been written. And the World Health Organization would not have declared a global tobacco epidemic.

Tobacco use produced about 3.1 million deaths worldwide in 1995 and will result in about 500 million premature deaths among the present world's population (Collishaw & Lopez, 1996). The active life of the cigarette has caused the early death of men and women, becoming, in the words of the surgeon general, "the most important preventable cause of death in our society" (U.S. Department of Health and Human Services [USDHHS], 1990). In the United States, eventually about half (1 in 2) of all tobacco users die of a smoking-related disease (Burns et al., 1997). As cigarettes spread among peoples of the world, other nations will bear similar costs of smoking. The World Bank (1993) has projected that "by the third decade [of the 21st century], smoking is expected to kill 10 million people annually worldwide—more than the total of deaths from malaria, maternal and major childhood conditions, and tuberculosis combined."

Who Smokes

A Worldview

The World Health Organization has been mobilizing to try to control the worldwide tobacco epidemic. Globally, almost half of all men (47%) and more than 1 in 10 women (12%) smoke (World Bank, 1999). More economically developed countries (e.g., United States, Sweden, France) have generally already been

TABLE 3.1 Smoking Prevalence Among Men and Women in 14 Selected Countries

Country	Year Surveyed	Male Prevalence %	Female Prevalence %
Republic of Korea (South Korea)	1989	68.2	6.7
Dominican Republic	1990	66.3	13.6
People's Republic of China	1984	61.0	7.0
Poland	1993	51.0	29.0
France	1993	40.0	27.0
Brazil	1989	39.9	25.4
Mexico	1990	38.3	14.4
Norway	1994	36.4	35.5
Canada	1991	31.0	29.0
Australia	1993	29.0	21.0
United Kingdom	1994	28.0	26.0
United States	1991	28.1	23.5
Nigeria	1990	24.4	6.7
Sweden	1994	22.0	24.0

SOURCE: World Health Organization (1996).

taking steps to reduce smoking. For males 15 and over, the percentage of daily smoking has declined in recent years to about 42% in the early 1990s; for females, the smoking prevalence was never as high as for males and was 24% in the early 1990s in more developed countries (Collishaw & Lopez, 1996). Less developed regions (e.g., India, China, Sub-Saharan Africa) have a higher smoking prevalence among males (47%) and a lower smoking prevalence for females (7%). On the basis of historical patterns, cigarette use will likely rise dramatically for females in less developed countries unless significant tobacco control measures are put in place. As cultural restrictions against smoking collapse, smoking consumption rises among women. The prevalence of tobacco use has been shifting from men in high-income regions to women in high-income regions and men in low-income regions (Mackay & Crofton, 1996; World Bank, 1999). See Table 3.1 for different patterns of recent prevalence figures in selected countries. Sweden has one of the lowest percentages of smoking for men and women, with slightly more women than men smoking. Korea has over 3 times the prevalence of male smoking than in Sweden. For females, in contrast, Korea has one third the prevalence of female smoking than in Sweden. If the smoking levels listed in Table 3.1 don't change, different countries will in the future have very different rates of smoking-caused disease in men and women and overall.

Smoking in the United States

Sex differences are decreasing. Figure 3.1 shows the dramatic rise of the cigarette in the United States in the 20th century along with indications of major events that seem to have influenced cigarette use. Much of the peak level of smoking is due to men. In the 1950s in the United States, the social pressures strongly supported smoking by men and discouraged smoking by women. Seventy percent of young men smoked and half as many young women (35%) smoked (USDHHS, 1980; Warner & Murt, 1982). At the present time in the United States, smoking prevalence for both males and females is below 30% and just a few percentage points apart (see Table 3.1).

The genetics of smoking, one of the biological factors involved in smoking, have not changed for men and women in the past 50 years. So the genetics of smoking cannot account for such a dramatic convergence in smoking prevalence. This is likely to be a largely cultural rather than biological effect. Local cultures, customs, and beliefs can determine who smokes and who does not.

"Better off" persons are less likely to smoke. Individuals with better jobs, higher incomes, and more years of education are said to have higher socioeconomic status. Socioeconomic status is a very important epidemiological measure. Persons with higher socioeconomic status generally have better health and live longer than do those with lower socioeconomic status (Adler et al., 1994). Figure 3.2 shows the prevalence of smoking for those who (a) didn't finish high school, (b) finished high school only, and (c) completed college as of 1966 and 1995. At both time points, twice as many smokers are in the low-education group than in the high-education group. About half as many smokers are found in each group in 1995 compared with 1966. This figure highlights the powerful interrelationships between time, socioeconomic status, and cigarette smoking.

Geographical variation within the United States. Given the mobility and diversity of current U.S. society, it is unlikely that inherent genetic or biological differences would make tobacco use more prevalent in one region than in another.

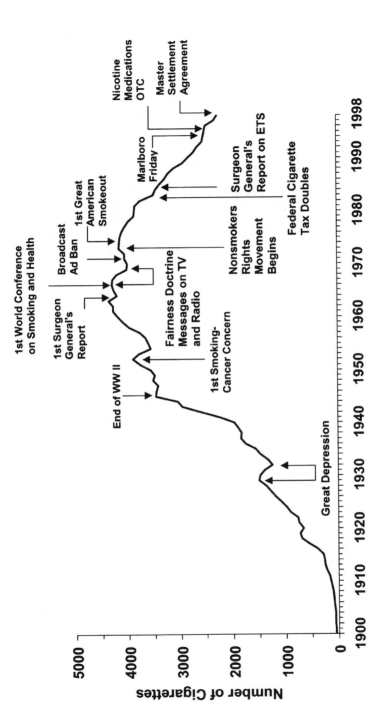

Figure 3.1. Adult per Capita Cigarette Consumption and Major Smoking and Health Events—United States, 1900-1998

SOURCE: Centers for Disease Control and Prevention.

35

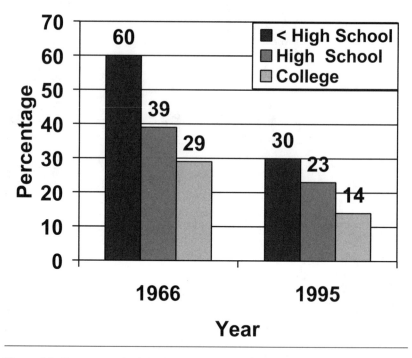

Figure 3.2. Percentage of Adult Cigarette Smokers in the United States in 1966 in 1995 among Those Who Had Less Than a High School Diploma, a High School Diploma, or a College Degree
SOURCE: Centers for Disease Control and Prevention.

However, the differences in tobacco use rates among states are dramatic. Utah has the lowest percentage of smokers: 13.3% (16.4% of males, 10.1% of females; Centers for Disease Control and Prevention [CDC], 1998a). Utah also has a significant proportion of residents whose religious beliefs prohibit the use of tobacco. This creates a cultural environment in which even those who are not members of that faith are most likely influenced by living in a place where tobacco use is discouraged. In California, 17.5% of males and 13.6% of females smoke. In November of 1988, the California government initiated an antismoking campaign and increased cigarette taxes, actions that have decreased tobacco sales and use. In contrast, Kentucky is a major tobacco-growing state, alone accounting for 27% of all U.S. tobacco production (Snell, 1999). Because tobacco is a major component of its economy, it is not surprising that tobacco use there is high. Kentucky is highest in overall adult smoking rates (33.1% of males, 28.7% of females). Nearly three times more women smoke in Kentucky than in Utah. Also, Kentucky has one of the highest rates of smokeless tobacco use among men (8.5%) (CDC, 2000b). Smokeless tobacco use among women and girls in the United States rarely equals that of boys and men. Kentucky can be predicted to have a much higher burden of tobacco-caused diseases than Utah.

What Kills Smokers

This chapter emphasizes the role of cigarettes in accounting for tobacco-related deaths. Smokeless tobacco products and uninhaled cigars or pipes are also dangerous and produce death and disability, although to a lesser extent. The modern cigarette is designed to be mild enough so that most smokers can inhale tobacco smoke into the lungs. Indeed, the great appeal of the cigarette derives from the consequences of its inhalability. With most cigarettes, noninhalation—just puffing and holding a cigarette in one's mouth—will not get enough nicotine to the brain to make smoking worthwhile for the smoker. Tobacco smoke in the lungs is the obvious perpetrator of lung cancer and the respiratory diseases of emphysema and bronchitis.

Lung Cancer: The First Epidemiological Evidence

Richard Doll, a young British medical researcher, was a smoker himself when he first began to reach the conclusion that tobacco was killing patients. He watched the hospital charts and death certificates of men in post-World War II England list lung cancer as a cause of illness and death. He soon saw smoking as "a mug's [fool's] game" and quit smoking in 1949. He went on to become one of a handful of scientists who identified tobacco as a significant health hazard, and he fired some of the first shots in what became a war against tobacco.

In an interview in 1999 at the age of 86 (Brown, 1999), Doll recalled that his father had offered to pay him the equivalent of 4 months' wages for an English workingman—if Doll would not smoke until age 21. His father, a physician, made the offer not in the interest of health, but because he saw tobacco as a waste of money. The younger Doll, however, started smoking anyway at age 18.

At that time, most men smoked, and no one in medical schools mentioned tobacco as a health hazard. Doll, a soldier with a French battalion in World War II, was forced to end his military career when he lost a kidney to tuberculosis. He came back to Britain when the country was in the midst of an unexplained epidemic of lung cancer that was also affecting Europe and the United States. When the British Medical Research Council first enlisted Doll to help find the cause of this epidemic, his best guess was that "it had something to do with motorcars." After he and statistician Bradford Hill examined interviews and diagnoses of patients at 20 London hospitals, they found a strong relationship between smoking and lung cancer.

Doll and Hill were prepared to publish these findings in 1949 but were asked by the Medical Research Council to conduct a parallel study at other hospitals. With parallel results, they published their findings (Doll & Hill, 1950). Doll and Hill then surveyed British doctors to identify those who smoked. Within 2.5 years, the physicians who smoked were dying of lung cancer—a finding that Doll and Hill published (Doll & Hill, 1954). Surprisingly, the Medical Research Council concluded by 1957 that it was unnecessary to fund further studies of smoking because it was now established that smoking caused lung cancer. For decades since then, the tobacco industry has disputed the claim that smoking causes cancer. The Doll and Hill work was important, but not sufficient to end all debate about smoking and health or answer all of the scientific questions on the matter. At the same time that Doll was evaluating the potential causes of lung cancer, young researcher Ernst L. Wynder at Washington University in St. Louis, Missouri, had been intrigued by his clinical observations of an apparent relationship between smoking and lung cancer. With little support from seemingly unconcerned colleagues, he persevered and began his pioneering epidemiological studies of the relationship between smoking and lung cancer. Even the American Cancer Society was initially uninterested, although ultimately that group did begin to fund the work that led to Wynder and Evarts Graham's publication of an article in the *Journal of the American Medical Association* (Wynder & Graham, 1950) on "tobacco smoking as a tentative etiological factor" in a type of cancer. Wynder followed up this work with further investigations in animals and humans, eventually leading him and others to conclude that cigarette smoking was indeed properly categorized as a cause of cancer.

Findings by Wynder, Doll, and their colleagues about tobacco spurred a movement toward tobacco cessation that is still thriving. In the United States, the rate of new cancer cases and deaths for all forms of cancer is continuing to decline, although an increase in adolescent smoking could reverse that trend. A 1999 report shows that the number of new cancer cases declined an average of just under 1% for each year from 1990 to 1996 (Wingo et al., 1999). This represented a reversal of a trend showing an increased rate from 1973 to 1990. Cancer deaths have been declining at a rate slightly slower than the decrease in the overall rate of new cases of cancer each year.

Establishing "Causation" in Epidemiology

Representatives of the cigarette industry have spoken repeatedly of the "smoking and health controversy," as if the scientific jury was still out on the matter. In 1967, the first warning printed on cigarettes in the United States did say: "Caution: Smoking *may be* [italics added] hazardous to your health." Nearly 30 years later, on April 14, 1994, the executives for the seven major cigarette manufacturers in the United States testified under oath in front of a committee of the House of Representatives in the public light of television cameras. Among the most remarkable testimony was *the assertion by each that smoking had not been proven to cause disease in humans.* For example, Andrew Tisch of Lorillard confirmed that he did not believe that cigarette smoking causes cancer. A key industry strategy has been to play on the public's misunderstanding and mistrust of statistics. For example, Mr. Tisch testified on April 14, 1996, that, "We have looked at the data and the data that we have been able to see has all been statistical data that has not convinced me that smoking causes death."

By 1997, Liggett Tobacco Company had broken ranks, acknowledging that smoking caused health problems, and by May of 2000, Lorillard and Brown & Williamson agreed. Remarkably, this still left the two largest cigarette manufacturers in the United States, Philip Morris and R. J. Reynolds, continuing to assert that cigarettes do not cause disease (Wilson, 2000).

If one looks at what was said over 30 years earlier at the time of the 1964 Smoking and Health Report of the surgeon general (U.S. Department of Health, Education and Welfare [USDHEW], 1964), one can see that the cigarette industry response has remained consistent and self-serving. From documents from and books on the cigarette industry (see Brecher, 1972; Glantz, Slade, Bero, Hananer, & Barnes, 1996; Kluger, 1996), it is clear that the industry has worked to throw doubt on the conclusions of the surgeon general.

It is justified scientifically that the rotating warnings on cigarette packs in the United States now include the statement, "Smoking Causes Lung Cancer, Heart

Disease, Emphysema, and May Complicate Pregnancy." It is important to understand the basis for such judgments about causation. To do that, it is necessary to understand the rules of epidemiological evidence.

In some sciences, causality can be proven conclusively by means of repeated, random-assignment experimentation. Such experimentation uses random selection of the groups studied to maximize the chances that the groups are not different from each other to begin with. If one wanted to know if a new type of fertilizer causes corn to grow taller than does an old type of fertilizer, how could one tell if any growth associated with the new fertilizer is caused by the fertilizer and not some preexisting differences in the growing potential of the soil in the field? One can select several fields at random (e.g., by flipping a coin) to receive either the new or the old fertilizer. If the fields using the new fertilizer grow taller corn than do the other fields, it is likely that the new fertilizer caused this extra growth.

However, it is not possible or ethical to select children at random to become smokers or nonsmokers. In the real world, individuals self-select to take up smoking or not, or to continue smoking or not. Maybe (probably) those who take up smoking are different in many ways from those who do not take up smoking. And maybe some of the preexisting ways in which smokers are different from non-smokers also represent characteristics that influence risks for disease. Thus, it would be impossible (or unethical) to design a random-assignment experiment to establish that smoking is not just *associated* with disease but results in disease. To require that actions be decided only on the basis of perfect proof—when the perfect experimental proof can never be attained—is an impractical position. To say that an *association* is not a *cause* until it has been experimentally proven in humans is to rig the game, so to speak, such that the cigarette industry cannot lose.

Epidemiologists and public health officials often make decisions based on imperfect evidence. Some of the most important questions are not subject to strict experimental tests. When scientists in the 1950s and 1960s were evaluating the health consequences of smoking, five special criteria were used to help determine when an association was the result of a causal relationship. It was acknowledged that "statistical methods cannot establish proof of a causal relationship" (USDHEW, 1964, p. 20) and that five additional criteria were necessary: (a) consistency of the association, (b) strength of the association, (c) specificity of the association, (d) temporal relationship of the association, and (e) coherence of association. It should also be noted that to conclude that smoking causes disease (e.g., lung cancer) is not to conclude that smoking is the only cause, but rather that it is one cause. Diseases are often the result of complex biobehavioral processes involving a number of causative factors.

Consistency of the association. A consistent association is one that is found repeatedly as well as one that is found using different techniques. If a relationship is not found over and over, it is probably not causal. If only one kind of study shows the relationship, the quirks of that study may be responsible for the observed association.

Strength of the association. Strength of association has been measured often with an epidemiological index called relative risk or the relative risk ratio. The occurrence of disease X among smokers (for example, in 30 of every 100) and the occurrence of disease X among nonsmokers (perhaps in 2 of every 100) would indicate that one has 15 times ($\frac{30}{2} = 15$) the chance of getting the disease if one is a smoker. In other words, the risk of disease X for smokers *relative* to the risk for nonsmokers is 15 times greater (i.e., the risk ratio or relative risk is 15). Another aspect of the strength of the association can be the dose-response characteristics of the relationship—an increase in response related to an increase in dose (e.g., heavier vs. lighter smoking). The evidence that those who smoke more are at greater risk of disease than those who smoke less has been used to establish the strength of the association. Lung cancer death rates are about 20 to 30 times higher in heavy smokers than in nonsmokers, indicating a dose-response relationship (USDHEW, 1979).

Specificity of the association. This criterion is related to the strength of the association. *Specificity* refers to identifying specific relationships between a possible causal agent and a specific disease. Cigarette smoke is complex, and some elements in smoke may be more related to cancer, whereas others may be more related to heart disease or to emphysema. To the extent that specific agents are related to specific diseases, a causal relationship is supported.

Temporal relationship of the association. The proposed cause of an effect needs to occur before the effect. Smoking-caused cancer needs to be found in individuals previously exposed to cigarettes.

Coherence of association. A coherent association is one that makes sense in terms of possible mechanisms for the effect. A dose-response relationship helps establish coherence. The specificity of an association may also suggest mechanisms by which the exposure would cause the disease.

These five criteria of association all point to smoking causing disease.

▦ Smoking Kills

Medieval scholarship has been ridiculed because of fruitless debates on how many angels can dance on the head of a pin. A smoking-versus-health controversy is not only similarly fruitless; it is dangerous. To reject the epidemiological evidence as unpersuasive is to help perpetuate the unrestrained use of a deadly product. Figure 3.1 suggests that the Smoking and Health Report of 1964 contributed to the decline of the cigarette. If public authorities had not declared smoking as a cause of death and disability in 1964, the public health burden of smoking would be even greater than it is today. It has been estimated that between 1964 and 1985, about 750,000 smoking-related deaths were avoided or postponed as a result of smokers' and potential smokers' decisions to quit or to not start smoking cigarettes; each one of these delayed deaths represents an average gain in life expectancy of 20 years (USDHHS, 1989).

Hardly a week passes without the announcement of new warnings about the health hazards of smoking tobacco. Lung cancer received early attention, because smoking greatly increases one's likelihood for developing the disease and lung cancer was rare before smoking was common. Many people are unaware that cardiovascular disorders (those involving the heart and circulatory system) are the most frequent health risk from cigarette smoking in the United States at the present time. The pattern of diseases related to the global smoking epidemic varies somewhat around the world. In China, for example, smoking-related respiratory disease is a more important cause of death than lung cancer (Collishaw & Lopez, 1996).

These are some common misconceptions about the health risks of using tobacco:

- ▪ *Misconception:* Cigars and smokeless tobaccos (spit tobacco, moist snuff) carry no risks of disease.
- ▪ *Misconception:* Smoking filtered, low-tar, and low-nicotine cigarettes carries less risk than smoking regular-strength cigarettes, particularly those without filters. (See Chapter 8 for more on this.)
- ▪ *Misconception:* Smoking is safe if a person doesn't smoke more than 10 or 15 cigarettes a day.
- ▪ *Misconception:* Smoking during pregnancy doesn't really hurt the baby.

These are all false notions. Smoking carries risks for the smoker and for others exposed to tobacco smoke. One large cigar can deliver many times the amounts of tar and nicotine to the smoker, as well as to exposed nonsmokers, as would be delivered from one cigarette. All forms of tobacco use expose users to dangerous toxins.

Studying Epidemiological Patterns

The more one uses tobacco, the greater the risk of dying from a smoking-caused disease. The relative risk for lung cancer, heart disease, and all-cause mortality (death from all causes) is a function of the amount smoked (i.e., there is a "coherent association"). Table 3.2 shows the patterns of relative risk as daily use of tobacco (cigars or cigarettes) increases.

Primary cigar smokers are those who have never smoked cigarettes. Secondary cigar smokers are former and current cigarette smokers. They are more likely to inhale cigar smoke than are primary cigar smokers, and this inhalation does bring greater risk of death. (Data for secondary cigar smokers are omitted from the table.) A relative risk of 1.00 would indicate that the users have no greater risk of death than do nonusers: If 10 in 100 users and 10 in 100 nonusers die, the relative risk would be 1.00 (i.e., $^{10}/_{10} = 1$); if 20 in 100 users and 10 in 100 nonusers die, the relative risk would be 2.00 (i.e., $^{20}/_{10} = 2$), meaning that 2 times as many users as nonusers die. The death rates per 100,000 are often calculated in studies that assess smoking habits and mortality. Studies differ in the number of persons studied, the age of the persons, the number of years studied, and the country or location of the study. Specific characteristics of the persons studied (like income and education level and health) will also influence the findings. Statistical testing is done to estimate the likelihood that the relative risk calculated in a particular study is reliably greater (or less than) 1.00. The 95% confidence limit refers to a range of relative risks that is likely to be found 95% of the time. If the confidence limits include the number 1, as is the case for all-cause death for cigar smokers who smoke only 1 to 2 cigars per day (see Table 3.2), then this analysis shows that these smokers experience no extra risk of death compared to nonsmokers. Although no one study is conclusive, the Cancer Prevention Survey 1 (Burns et al., 1997) provides a good example of the magnitude of smoking risks.

In Table 3.2, the relative risk for lung cancer (e.g., 20.23 for smokers of 21 or more cigarettes per day) is much higher than the relative risk for coronary heart disease (e.g., 1.65 for smokers of 21 or more cigarettes per day). Why might this be the case? Look at the number of deaths observed for these two groups (see Table 3.2). Note how many more individuals die of coronary heart disease than of lung cancer. Many people who have never smoked die from heart disease, because

TABLE 3.2 Relative Risk Ratios for Death From Coronary Heart Disease,[a] Cancer of the Lung/Bronchus, and All Causes, by Level of Cigar/Cigarettes Per Day From Cancer Prevention Study [1]

Daily Use	Coronary Heart Disease Relative Risk (95%CL)	Coronary Heart Disease Deaths[b]	Cancer, Lung, and Bronchus Relative Risk (95%CL)	Cancer, Lung, and Bronchus Deaths[b]	All Cause Mortality Relative Risk (95%CL)	All Cause Deaths[b]
Primary cigar						
1-2	0.98 (0.91,1.07)	1,505/8,202	0.9 (0.54,1.66)	73/191	1.02 (0.97,1.07)	3,698/19,667
3-4	1.06 (0.96,1.16)		2.36 (1.49,3.54)		1.08 (1.02,1.15)	
5+	1.14 (1.03,1.24)		3.40 (2.34,4.77)		1.17 (1.10,1.24)	
Combined	1.05 (1.00-1.11)		2.10 (1.63,2.65)		1.08 (1.05,1.12)	
Cigarette only						
1-19	1.40 (1.36,1.45)	15,659/8,202	6.75 (6.18,7.37)	3,166/191	1.46 (1.43,1.49)	38,220/19,667
20	1.58 (1.54,1.62)		12.86 (12.14,13.60)		1.69 (1.66,1.71)	
21+	1.65 (1.58,1.62)		20.23 (19.20,21.90)		1.88 (1.85,1.91)	
Combined	1.54 (1.52,1.57)		12.39 (11.97,12.83)		1.66 (1.64,1.68)	

SOURCE: Based on numbers from the CPS-1 Study (National Cancer Institute, 1997).

NOTE: Age-standardized rate ratio for smoking group compared to never-smokers. Primary cigar smokers have never smoked cigarettes and are unlikely to inhale.

a. With 95% confidence limits.

b. Number of deaths in subject group/never-smoker group.

smoking is not the only cause of heart disease; few nonsmokers die of lung cancer, because smoking is a leading cause of lung cancer. Note that although many smokers are very concerned about the lung cancer risks of smoking, many more smokers will die of coronary heart disease. A large relative risk can indicate a strong causative agent, but it does not necessarily indicate the largest public health issue.

Lung cancer, which causes 28% of all cancer deaths, more deaths than any other cancer, is a key factor driving overall cancer rates. Active smoking and exposure to environmental tobacco smoke are believed to cause about 90% of all lung cancer cases. Although lung cancer rates are decreasing among men of most ethnic and racial groups, lung cancer rates are increasing among women, reflecting previous increases in smoking by women. Since 1987, lung cancer has surpassed breast cancer as a cause of death in women (CDC, 1993).

Some 52% of male smoker deaths and 43% of female smoker deaths can be attributed to tobacco use (Burns et al., 1997). Tobacco use is a cause of or contributing factor to over 400,000 deaths per year in the United States (USDHHS, 1990). Table 3.3 presents those deaths from diseases related to smoking. An average smoker has about 10 times the risk of lung cancer and 2 times the risk of cardiovascular disease as a nonsmoker has. Smoking increases the risk of contracting and dying from lung cancer more than from cardiovascular disease, but more smokers die from coronary heart disease than from lung cancer.

Nor do the statistics stop with heart disease and lung cancer. The following medical conditions can be caused or exacerbated by tobacco use:

- *Cardiovascular:* peripheral vascular disease, coronary heart disease, angina pectoris, heart attack, arrhythmia, cardiomyopathy, aneurysm
- *Cancer:* lung, esophageal, laryngeal, bladder, oral, kidney, stomach, pancreatic, cervical, vulvar, colorectal
- *Senses:* vision impairment, hearing impairment
- *Respiratory:* chronic obstructive lung disease, asthma, respiratory infections
- *Skin:* premature wrinkling, palmoplantar pustulosis, psoriasis
- *Bones:* degeneration of discs in back, musculoskeletal injury
- *Rheumatoid:* Arthritis and osteoporosis
- *Reproduction:* pregnancy and delivery difficulties, low birth-weight infants, birth defects, cognitively and behaviorally impaired offspring

TABLE 3.3 Cigarette Smoking-Related Mortality in the United States, 1996

Disease	Men	Women	Overall
Cancers			
Lung	81,179	35,741	116,920
Lung from ETS	1,055	1,945	3,000
Other	21,659	9,743	31,402
Total	103,893	47,429	151,322
Cardiovascular diseases			
Hypertension	3,233	2,151	5,450
Heart disease	88,644	45,591	134,235
Stroke	14,978	8,303	23,281
Other	11,682	5,172	16,854
Total	118,603	61,117	179,820
Respiratory diseases			
Pneumonia	11,292	7,881	19,173
Bronchitis/emphysema	9,234	5,541	14,865
Chronic airway obstruction	30,385	18,579	48,982
Other	787	668	1,455
Total	51,788	32,689	84,475
Diseases among infants	1,006	705	1,711
Burn deaths	863	499	1,362
All causes	276,153	142,537	418,690

SOURCE: Office on Smoking and Health (1996).

How do such health risks happen? Consider the case of tobacco-caused coronary heart disease, which kills some 90,000 persons in the United States each year. Nicotine, the addictive agent of tobacco smoke, mimics the effects of the sympathetic nervous system (Benowitz, 1998a). Smoking increases a person's heart rate by as much as 30% during the first few minutes after smoking. Circulating catecholamines (hormones involved in the stress response, such as adrenaline) increase during smoking (Benowitz, 1998b). Blood pressure rises as blood vessels constrict, forcing the heart to work harder to deliver oxygen to the body. At the same time, the carbon monoxide from tobacco smoke competes with oxygen to bind to hemoglobin in the blood (carbon monoxide has a higher affinity for hemoglobin than oxygen), limiting the capacity of the blood to deliver oxygen to the tissues (Benowitz, 1998b). Consequently, the heart must work much harder than it would otherwise.

Smoking tends to result in higher overall blood pressure, as well as in greater swings in blood pressure. Tobacco smoking also appears to contribute to atherosclerosis, a condition in which the arteries are clogged and narrowed by the accumulation of fatty substances and tissues in the arterial lining (Benowitz, 1998b). Nicotine renders the blood hypercoagulable (i.e., more able to clot) by activating platelets, increasing the risk for thrombosis (clotting inside the blood vessels) (Benowitz, 1998b). Smokers are also less likely to respond well to treatment for clearing arteries clogged by atherosclerosis.

These conditions place smokers at increased risk for myocardial infarction (heart attack), a condition in which some part of the heart muscle does not receive adequate oxygen, resulting in muscle death. Acute thrombosis of the type described above is highly associated with myocardial infarction (Benowitz, 1998b). The risk of myocardial infarction among current smokers is about three times higher than among nonsmokers (USDHHS, 1990).

▓ Health Risks of
Other Tobacco Products

Because the body absorbs tobacco in different ways through different routes of administration, the health risks also vary. It is not surprising, then, that one form of tobacco results in health risks that differ from risks associated with another form. For example, users of moist oral snuff (the most popular type of smokeless or spit tobacco) have a somewhat greater chance of developing oral cancer (relative risk = 4.0) than do cigarette smokers (USDHHS, 1986). And cigarette smokers have a greater chance of developing lung cancer than do snuff users.

Even low levels of tobacco use can be dangerous and can result in disease. Smoking only a few cigarettes a day is less dangerous than heavier smoking, although the reality is that few smokers can limit themselves to a few cigarettes a day, regardless of their intentions when they first begin smoking. Part of the hazard of tobacco use is that it compounds other health risks one might not recognize. As an example, someone who uses both alcohol and tobacco has a dramatically increased risk of esophageal cancer (e.g., USDHEW, 1979)—the whole of alcohol and tobacco risks is more that the sum of its parts.

Smokeless Tobacco

Smokeless tobacco has been rising in popularity, particularly among male high school students (CDC, 1998b, 1998c). A dentist or dental hygienist may be the first person to discover that a snuff user is developing health problems related to tobacco use. An early condition called "snuff dipper's lesion" is marked by reversible changes in the epithelium (USDHHS, 1986). Recession of gingiva (gums) and discoloration of teeth also can be attributed to the use of smokeless tobacco, although these typically do not reverse when snuff use is discontinued (USDHHS, 1986). Smokeless tobacco (particularly moist snuff) users develop oral cancer at a rate 7 times that of nonusers; evidence for association with other cancers is sparse and inconclusive at best (Bolinder, 1997; USDHHS, 1986). Smokeless tobacco also increases heart rates and may increase the incidence of cardiovascular disease (USDHHS, 1986). A dose-response relationship exists for many of the health effects—the more smokeless tobacco used the greater the risk for disease (USDHHS, 1986). Clearly, the health risks of smokeless tobacco should not be dismissed or taken lightly.

Cigars

Cigar smoking exploded in popularity in the United States beginning in the early 1990s, coinciding with increased promotion of their use (CDC, 1997; Burns, 1998). Within 5 years, billions of cigars were consumed annually in the United States, and the NCI responded with a comprehensive monograph in 1998 detailing the health effects of cigars.

Cigar smoking generally differs from cigarette smoking in that the smoke does not need to be inhaled for nicotine absorption to occur, because cigar smoke is more alkaline than cigarette smoke (see Chapter 4). However, inhalation of cigar smoke is much more common in those who switch from cigarettes to cigars, or those who smoke both cigars and cigarettes (Burns, 1998). Cigar (and cigarette) smokers can accurately report if they inhale or not, but reports of "depth of inhalation" are not as valuable (Herling & Kozlowski, 1988). The disease risks associated with cigars differ from those associated with cigarettes, even though both are smoked tobacco products. The results in Table 3.2 show that, compared with nonsmokers, cigar users' relative risks are about 8 for oral cancer, 2 for lung cancer, and 7 for buccal and pharyngeal cancers. The relative risk for lung cancer rises significantly for cigar smokers who inhale or smoke more than 1 to 2 cigars per day, as well as for secondary cigar smokers (NCI, 1998). It is now clear that cigars are not necessarily safer than cigarettes but that those who smoke at low rates, start smoking later in life, and do not regularly inhale appear to be at lower risks of disease than are those who started younger and smoked heavier (Baker et al., 2000). One series of studies found that the risk of disease was similar in smokers of cigarettes, pipes, and cigars if the users were inhaling similar amounts of smoke (Wald & Watt, 1997).

Cancer is not the sole risk of cigar smoking. Those who smoke many cigars per day and those who inhale are at a greater risk (relative risks = 1.14 and 1.37, respectively) for coronary heart disease (Burns, 1998). Cigar smokers who inhale also are 4.5 times more likely to develop chronic obstructive pulmonary disease. However, those cigar smokers who do not inhale directly are still likely to be exposed to secondhand cigar smoke.

Passive Exposure to Tobacco Smoke

The toxic components found in mainstream cigarette smoke (i.e., what the smoker inhales) are also found in secondhand smoke, sometimes in higher concentrations (USDHHS, 1989). Measurable levels of cotinine (the primary metabolite of nicotine) can be found in up to 88% of nonsmokers (CDC, 1993). Until recently, smoking was permitted in most public and private buildings, and exposure to environmental tobacco smoke was widespread in the United States.

Evidence suggests that children and nonsmoking adults can become the victims of some of the same medical conditions that afflict smokers. Nonsmokers who are routinely exposed to environmental tobacco smoke are at increased risk (relative risk = 1.3) of lung cancer (USDHHS, 1989). They also have a 30% greater risk of serious cardiovascular disease (NCI, 1999). There is also inconsistent evidence that secondhand smoke exposure is associated with cancers of the breast, cervix, bladder, and leukemia, although more study is needed in this area (NCI, 1999). Asthma symptoms in adults and children can be worsened by exposure to secondhand smoke. Furthermore, evidence suggests that secondhand smoke can cause asthma in children; in California, between 1,000 and 3,000 new cases of asthma per year have been linked to smoke exposure (NCI, 1999).

Infants in households where someone smokes are at almost twice the risk for sudden infant death syndrome (SIDS; NCI, 1999). Children of smokers suffer twice as many respiratory infections as children of nonsmokers (NCI, 1999). Other data have been published linking secondhand smoke exposure to myriad negative prenatal health outcomes (e.g., spontaneous abortion, malformation); however, these data are weak at best (NCI, 1999).

These risks led the Environmental Protection Agency to label tobacco smoke a Class A carcinogen (i.e., a known human carcinogen) in 1993. The knowledge that secondhand smoke can be dangerous has been a primary catalyst in the massive movement against cigarette smoking.

Summary

Smoking is a major cause of premature death and disability worldwide. The World Bank has projected that "by the third decade [of the 21st century], smoking is expected to kill 10 million people annually worldwide—more than the total of deaths from malaria, maternal and major childhood conditions, and tuberculosis combined" (World Bank, 1993). The percentage of smokers varies substantially within the United States and elsewhere around the world. Psychosocial and cultural factors seem responsible for dramatic differences in tobacco use as a function of gender, socioeconomic status, and geographical region. Many smoking-caused diseases occur after many years of smoking. Cardiovascular disease, lung cancer, other cancers, emphysema, and other respiratory diseases are increased by tobacco use. Those who don't smoke themselves but who are chronically exposed to cigarette smoke also appear to be at increased risk of disease. The relative importance of smoking-caused diseases varies somewhat from country to country.

Further Reading

National Cancer Institute. (1997). *Changes in cigarette-related disease risks and their implication for prevention and control.* D. M. Burns, L. Garfinkel, & J. M. Samet (Eds.) Bethesda, MD: National Cancer Institute.

This monograph provides an excellent review of epidemiological evidence, with an emphasis on the United States.

World Bank. (1999). *Curbing the epidemic: Governments and the economics of tobacco control.* Washington, DC: Author.

This report provides an international perspective on tobacco and health.

4

What Nicotine Does to the Body

*Think of the cigarette as a dispenser for a dose unit of
nicotine . . . Think of a puff of smoke as a vehicle for
nicotine . . . Smoke is beyond question the most optimized
vehicle of nicotine and the cigarette the most optimized
dispenser of smoke.*

—William Dunn, Senior Researcher for Philip Morris
Company(1972) as quoted in Hurt and Robertson (1998)

Two thousand degrees Fahrenheit. From the microblast furnace core of the burning cigarette, nicotine is vaporized and freed to quickly enter the body through the lung. Racing with the blood, it reaches the brain faster and affects the rest of the body more readily than could be achieved by intravenous injection. Even when delivered to the body by way of chewing tobacco or snuff, nicotine's chemical properties allow it to be very rapidly absorbed into the bloodstream. Within seconds of puffing on a cigarette or a few minutes of "dipping" snuff, the user feels the effects of nicotine. These effects can be detected by objective measurement of a variety of physical reactions, including brain function. This chapter will review the effects of nicotine on the body.

History

Nicotine had a crucial role in 20th-century research on physiology and in the development of modern neuropharmacology (Swedberg, Henningfield, & Goldberg, 1990). Studies at the beginning of the 20th century showed that nicotine activated certain muscle groups, that repeated application of nicotine led to diminished effects (tolerance), and that simultaneous application of chemicals such as curare (a nicotine antagonist) could block the effects of nicotine. Such research by John Langley and his colleagues led to Langley's (1906) postulation that some sort of "receptive substance" in tissues of the body responded differentially upon application of different chemicals. Langley's pioneering studies, which involved nicotine and other chemicals that had certain effects in common (e.g., strychnine) or that blocked the effects of nicotine (e.g., curare), were fundamental in mapping and exploring the nervous system (Lefkowitz, Hoffman, & Taylor, 1996). This research on nicotine also formed the basis for the modern *receptor theory* of drug action. Later, a branch of the peripheral nervous system was called the *nicotinic cholinergic system* because it was mapped by application of nicotine to various sites within the body. In the latter quarter of the 20th century, the pace of research on the pharmacological actions of nicotine progressed at a breathtaking pace, with hundreds of papers published every year, all of them reinforcing these basic findings about nicotine.

What Is Nicotine?

Tobacco is a plant with leaves that could be eaten except for the distaste and discomfort produced by the presence of the alkaloid nicotine. Alkaloids are plant-based organic chemicals such as cocaine, morphine, and quinine, which are generally basic or alkaline, meaning they have a pH in excess of 7 (Hoffman & Hoffman, 1997). Many alkaloids have been used either for their medicinal or poisonous qualities or for both. Nicotine is a tiny molecule that dissolves in both fatty and water-based substances (see Figure 4.1). This enables it to be rapidly absorbed through the skin and carried through the bloodstream to target receptors of the nervous system and organs (Balfour & Fagerstrom, 1996; Benowitz, 1996).

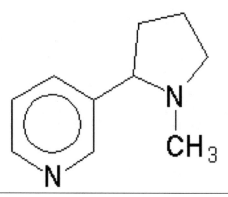

Figure 4.1. Nicotine's Chemical Structure

Most tobacco plants contain about 1% to 4% nicotine (Hoffman & Hoffman, 1997). Nicotine occurs in greater concentrations in the leaves than in the stems and stalks of the plant. Some hybrid tobacco plants have low levels of nicotine, and some have higher levels exceeding 6%. Thus, cigarettes, which typically use less than 1 gram of tobacco, contain about 10 mg of nicotine with a range of about 9 to 13 mg. Cigarette smokers generally get about 1 to 2 mg nicotine from each cigarette, with the rest either being left in the tobacco butt or going up in smoke.

Other tobacco products vary widely in their content and delivery of nicotine. For example, some cigars tested contained approximately 10 to more than 300 mg of nicotine each (Henningfield, Fant, Radzius, & Frost, 1999). Larger cigars tended to have more nicotine than smaller cigars, but the relationship was approximate. A typical 2 mg "plug" of smokeless tobacco ranges from a few milligrams of nicotine to more than 20 mg.

The amount of nicotine in tobacco may not seem like much, but nicotine is very potent. *Potency* refers to the amount of a drug it takes to produce a given effect—the smaller the amount of drug needed to produce the effect, the more potent the drug. Nicotine is 5 to 10 times more potent than cocaine or morphine in producing psychoactive (psychologically active) effects in humans or modifying behavior in animals (Henningfield, Schuh, & Jarvik, 1995; Swedberg et al., 1990).

Nicotine produces strong effects at higher doses and speeds of delivery. For example, nicotine, like cocaine and morphine, can be lethal at high doses and has been used as a pesticide. Nicotine can also reduce pain, although no dose of nicotine can reduce pain as well as morphine. Thus, on the measure of *analgesia* (pain reduction or absence), morphine is stronger than nicotine. On the other hand, daily doses of nicotine, which are associated with little discernable psychoactive effect, can reduce body weight and appetite. Cigarettes deliver nicotine in such a way that it reaches the brain and other target organs very rapidly in very high doses (Benowitz, 1996; Henningfield, Stapleton, Benowitz, & London, 1993).

■ Absorption of Nicotine in the Body

Popular tobacco products are convenient devices that allow people to consume controlled doses of nicotine (Slade, 1993). Tobacco products put nicotine into smoke or saliva, which allows its absorption into the bloodstream through the lungs as well as through the lining of the mouth, nose, and throat (Benowitz, 1996).

Inhalation of nicotine in smoke is the most rapid and efficient way to deliver nicotine (Benowitz, 1996). After nicotine is carried to the lungs by smoke, the lung's *alveoli* (air cells) enable the lungs to function as giant funnels to extract nicotine quickly and condense it into the pulmonary vein in a concentrated dose sometimes called the *bolus* (or lump). This concentrated dose of nicotine moves from the lungs to the left ventricle of the heart, where it is pumped through the arteries to the body. The small size of nicotine molecules along with their high degree of solubility in both water and fat enable nicotine to pass quickly through the membrane shield, called the *blood-brain barrier*, separating the brain from circulating blood (Henningfield, Schuh, & Jarvik, 1995; Hoffman & Hoffman, 1997). Thus, nicotine can reach the brain within 7 to 10 seconds from the time smoke is inhaled (Benowitz, 1996). This is the same process by which the body extracts oxygen from each breath of air and delivers oxygen throughout the body and brain (Henningfield et al. 1993). Ironically, the absorption and distribution of drugs such as nicotine, cocaine, and heroin occur through the same pathways and systems as the absorption and distribution of life-giving oxygen. Thus, this aspect of physiology that is so critical to the life-sustaining oxygenation of tissues can be hijacked by such drugs and thereby used to heighten their addictive actions.

Nicotine is absorbed more slowly when it is delivered by way of the mouth instead of the lungs. For example, smokeless tobacco placed in the mouth takes 10 to 20 minutes to achieve nicotine blood levels typically reached within just a few minutes of cigarette smoking (Benowitz, 1996; Hoffman & Hoffman, 1997)

The nicotine from cigarette smoke, which in this form has a pH of 6.0 to 7.0, is poorly absorbed if it is kept in the mouth (Hoffman & Hoffman, 1997). It must be inhaled deeply into the lungs, where absorption is rapid regardless of pH. This means that the particulate matter, gasses, and other toxins that make up cigarette smoke are also deeply inhaled into the lungs with each puff. Cigar smoke, which typically has a pH of 7 to 8, is effectively absorbed through the lining of the mouth. For this reason, it is not necessary for cigar smokers to inhale to obtain substantial doses of nicotine. However, cigar smokers who seek more rapid effects, particularly those who have also smoked cigarettes, often do inhale at least some smoke (Baker et al., 2000).

The principles of pH and nicotine absorption are applied in the making and marketing of some smokeless tobacco products (Connolly, 1995). Those products targeted to beginning users, so-called starter products, tend to have lower percentages of a form of nicotine that is readily absorbed, so less nicotine is available to the body. In contrast, the smokeless products preferred by more experienced users have a higher pH and deliver enough nicotine to make inexperienced users very nauseated on initial use but allow practiced users to obtain the high nicotine dosage levels to which they are accustomed.

It takes only 5 to 10 seconds for blood from the heart to reach most parts of the body, replenishing the body with oxygen through the arterial bloodstream. Blood is returned via the bloodstream, at a similar speed, to the right side of the heart, where it is pumped through the alveoli. There it releases carbon dioxide, carbon monoxide, and other substances (for smokers, this includes traces of nicotine) to be carried out of the body by each expired breath. While passing through the lungs, blood also absorbs fresh oxygen and other inhaled substances. Approximately once each minute, the entire blood supply is pumped through the heart. For smokers, this process rapidly distributes and dilutes the nicotine taken in with each puff of smoke (Benowitz, 1996; Henningfield et al., 1993).

Figure 4.2 shows how these factors affect nicotine absorption. Nicotine is absorbed rapidly following the inhalation of cigarette smoke and less rapidly through skin application in the form of a transdermal patch. Note also that the initial arterial levels of nicotine from inhaled cigarette smoke are 6 to 10 times higher than the venous levels shown in Figure 4.2 (American Psychiatric Association, 1996; Henningfield et al., 1993).

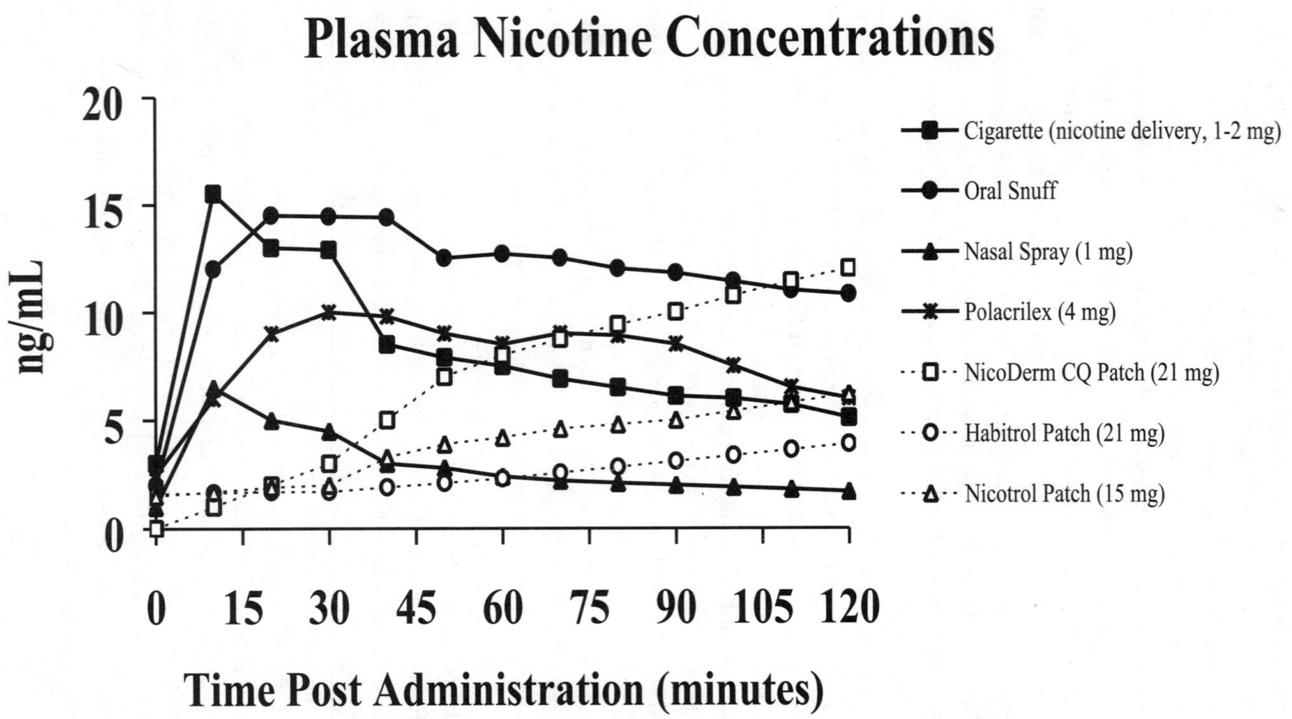

Plasma Nicotine Concentrations

Figure 4.2. Venous Blood Concentrations (in nanograms of nicotine per milliliter of blood) as a Function of Time for Various Nicotine Delivery Systems

■ How Long Does Nicotine Remain in the Body?

Within a few minutes of the time a cigarette is smoked, the high concentrations of nicotine in the arterial blood supply are redistributed into venous blood and diluted by about 90%. By this time, the nicotine bolus has disappeared and the nicotine levels in arterial and venous blood are about equal and will remain so until another cigarette is smoked. As the blood continues to circulate, nicotine is redistributed throughout the body, with higher concentrations left in areas such as the brain and liver, some transferred into urine by the kidneys, and some absorbed into fatty tissues. As a result of the redistribution phase, venous blood levels of nicotine decline by about 50% over the next 10 to 30 minutes. This is often referred to as the *initial half-life* or *redistribution half-life* of nicotine (i.e., the time it takes for the initial blood levels of nicotine to reduce by half).

The body can produce chemical changes in nicotine that break it down and turn it into different chemicals. In the 1980s, a series of studies by Neal Benowitz and others at the University of San Francisco demonstrated that the initial redistribution phase of nicotine was followed by a slower rate of falling blood levels, which was explained largely by nicotine metabolism (Benowitz, 1996). During this phase, blood levels decline by 50% approximately every 2 hours. Most of the metabolism occurs in the liver, although a small percentage of nicotine is also metabolized in the lungs and other organs.

During metabolism, most nicotine is converted to a substance called *cotinine* and to other chemicals that are much less potent and biologically active than nicotine (Benowitz, 1996). Cotinine has a half-life of about 20 hours and is easily measured in blood, urine, and saliva. This makes cotinine a convenient and reliable marker of how much nicotine a tobacco user has consumed, because cotinine levels do not rise and fall as quickly as nicotine levels do.

About 10% to 20% of nicotine is excreted unchanged in urine (Benowitz, 1996). The excretion is slightly faster if the urine is acidified (e.g., by consumption of vitamin C), and slightly slower if the urine is alkalinized (e.g., by consumption of antacids such as sodium bicarbonate). Schachter et al. (1977) found that increased acidification of the urine led to increased cigarette smoking and that increased stress produced increased urinary acidification. This may explain one of the reasons why addicted smokers smoke more under stress—to try to maintain nicotine levels to avoid withdrawal rather than because nicotine helps them cope (Silverstein, Kelly, Swan, & Kozlowski, 1982). Some people in the 1970s and 1980s suggested that smokers might reduce their tobacco consumption by taking antacids (Fix et al., 1983). However, the difference in excretion rates is so small between normal pH and alkalinized pH that the effect of antacid consumption on the elimination of nicotine is negligible (Grunberg & Kozlowski, 1986). Ironically, manipulating urinary pH has greater effects on increasing smoking than on decreasing smoking.

■ Pharmacodynamics:
Effects of Nicotine on the Body

As nicotine passes by certain nerve terminals and organs, it binds to bits of protein called *receptors* (Balfour & Fagerstrom, 1996). Some of these receptors are termed *nicotinic cholinergic* receptors because they were originally characterized as the subpopulation of receptors normally responding to acetyl*choline* and to nicotine (Lefkowitz, Hoffman, & Taylor, 1996). The receptors depolarize and send their electrical current to target organs. These receptors can activate skeletal muscles, trigger the release of *catecholamines* (biologically active chemicals that affect the body) such as *epinephrine* and *norepinephrine* from the adrenal gland, and release a biochemical called *dopamine* in the brain (Balfour & Fagerstrom, 1996; Benowitz, 1996).

Dramatic effects may follow, particularly if the person has had little prior contact with nicotine or if the dose is significantly larger than that to which the person is accustomed. For example, upon initial exposure to nicotine, the body typically reacts violently, as it might to other nerve poisons. The heart races, and the person may become intoxicated, delusional, light-headed, and nauseated and may even vomit (Benowitz, 1996; Henningfield et al., 1995). This extreme reaction rarely lasts more than a few hours, although farmers exposed to high doses of nicotine in pesticides can require a day or more of hospitalization.

With the first exposure of nicotine, the body begins to defend itself. Nicotine-rich beds in certain parts of the nervous system and brain grow (or *express*) more nicotine receptors to enable greater capacity for handling these toxic doses of nicotine (Balfour & Fagerstrom, 1996). With repeated nicotine exposure, toxicity gives way to *tolerance* and *addiction* (Swedberg et al., 1990).

Tolerance refers to adaptation to repeated drug exposure, such that the response diminishes as the person is repeatedly exposed to the drug (Benowitz, 1996; Swedberg et al., 1990). Over time, tolerance is often accompanied by increased intake of the drug to attain the same effects initially occurring at lower doses. However, tolerance differs for nicotine's varying effects and is not necessarily consistent across time. For example, the psychoactive effects and heart rate increase of nicotine use are strongest with the first few cigarettes of the day. Throughout the day, a smoker may respond very little to each additional cigarette, but each dose of nicotine continues to prevent the onset of withdrawal symptoms. However, abruptly increasing the dose will increase heart rate and yield some psychoactive effect.

Some tolerance dissipates after several hours of tobacco abstinence (Benowitz, 1996). Tobacco users awake each morning more sensitive to the effects of nicotine than they were when they went to sleep the night before (Balfour & Fagerstrom, 1996; Pillitteri, Kozlowski, Sweeney, & Heatherton, 1997). They report that the first few cigarettes of the day are among the best and most needed cigarettes. In fact, one of the single best indicators of nicotine dependence is how soon a smoker has the first cigarette after waking up each day (Kozlowski, Porter, Orleans, Pope, & Heatherton, 1994)

The tolerance of the nervous system to nicotine exposure has been studied since the beginning of the 20th century. The body uses several physiologic mechanisms in developing nicotine tolerance, including decreased responsiveness to the drug. This is termed *pharmacodynamic tolerance.* Although many people have assumed that experienced tobacco users metabolize nicotine more quickly than nonusers, research in the 1980s and 1990s suggested that this is not a reliable effect and that it is probably not the main mechanism by which tolerance develops (Benowitz, 1996).

Experienced tobacco users rarely experience a repetition of the profound nausea and sickness that may have accompanied their first use of tobacco. This appears to reflect some lasting tolerance, as well as a learned response of avoiding doses that are higher than they can withstand.

Tolerance may contribute to the long-term toxic effects of tobacco use. First, tolerance to nicotine permits users to take in greater quantities of tobacco-laden toxins than if they were still highly sensitive to small doses of nicotine. This increases their health risk, because people who smoke 25 cigarettes per day are at higher risk of tobacco-related disease than people who smoke fewer than 5 cigarettes per day. Also, tolerance leads to physical dependence, which not only permits people to consume high doses of nicotine but requires them to continue their intake at that level, lest they experience *withdrawal symptoms* (Balfour & Fagerstrom, 1996; Henningfield et al., 1995). After several weeks of nicotine exposure, physical dependence can develop. Nicotine-dependent persons then function normally when under the influence of nicotine but may report feeling abnormal or out of sorts when deprived of nicotine for more than a few hours (American Psychiatric Association, 1996; Balfour & Fagerstrom, 1996; Henningfield et al.,

1995). After quitting smoking, the person many experience these *withdrawal* or *abstinence systems* for weeks or months. These feelings are more than just the psychological distress of not holding a cigarette or not tasting smoke and inhaling it into the lungs. Nicotine products such as nicotine gum and patches can relieve these symptoms to some extent (Balfour & Fagerstrom, 1996; Henningfield et al., 1995; Fiore et al., 2000).

Physical dependence develops in most smokers while they are still in their youth. In fact, studies published by the Centers for Disease Control and Prevention (1994) indicate that young people experience withdrawal symptoms consistent with their heavy or light use of tobacco. Withdrawal symptoms are not *always* the strongest in those who use the most tobacco, but they are stronger on average (Henningfield et al., 1995). The ability of people to manage withdrawal symptoms when they quit smoking depends both on the severity of the symptoms and a person's capacity to manage pain and discomfort. (The withdrawal syndrome is described in Chapter 6.)

Reinforcement

Nicotine exposure directly activates mechanisms of reinforcement in the brain that reinforce behavior (Balfour & Fagerstrom, 1996; Swedberg et al., 1990). This is due, at least in part, to the ability of nicotine to increase dopamine levels in regions of the brain where reinforcement effects occur for other substances and responses (Royal College of Physicians, 2000). Thus, even healthy animals that are not physically dependent on nicotine will modify their behavior for doses of nicotine (Swedberg et al., 1990). Laboratory rats and monkeys will press levers many times to get small doses of nicotine that are delivered intravenously. Such laboratory experiments are termed *self-administration tests* and are a strong source of evidence that a drug is addictive. In the early 1980s, tobacco industry researcher Victor DeNoble demonstrated that rats would self-administer intravenous injections of nicotine (Kessler et al., 1996). His work was reviewed by his scientific peers and accepted for publication, but before it could be published, his employer made him retract his papers and closed his laboratory (Kessler et al., 1996). It wasn't until the late 1980s that other researchers independently discovered that rats made excellent subjects for studying the addictive properties of nicotine (Corrigall, 1999; Stolerman, 1999).

Humans find nicotine reinforcing and pleasurable (Henningfield et al., 1995; Stolerman, 1999). Studies by Henningfield and his colleagues in the 1980s showed that drug abusers frequently mistake injections of nicotine for amphetamine or cocaine (Henningfield et al., 1985). Although the drug abusers reported liking the effects of nicotine, they said they preferred to obtain nicotine through tobacco products, which allowed them to regulate their own doses. Even though many users initially find the taste, smell, and burn of tobacco unpleasant, the repeated, frequent pairing or association of these properties with the reinforcing effects of nicotine also makes those properties reinforcing (Henningfield et al., 1995; Stolerman, 1999).

Another way that tobacco use is reinforcing is in its capacity to alleviate the unpleasant and often intolerable withdrawal symptoms (Balfour & Fagerstrom, 1996; Henningfield et al., 1995). More than two thirds of cigarette smokers who try to quit relapse back to smoking within two days, unable to outlast the period during which the symptoms are at their peak. This does not mean that relapse to smoking is perfectly correlated with the worst of the withdrawal symptoms or that avoiding withdrawal symptoms is the only reason people smoke. The relationship between nicotine use and withdrawal is complicated. Nonetheless, nicotine withdrawal symptoms are widely accepted as a source of pressure for tobacco users to continue tobacco use, and alleviation of withdrawal symptoms is one means of helping smokers achieve and sustain abstinence (Balfour & Fagerstrom, 1996; Henningfield, 1995).

Other Nicotine-Based Reasons for Smoking

In addition to nicotine's reinforcing properties and its ability to curb withdrawal symptoms, tobacco users also find that nicotine provides other reasons for continued use (Balfour & Fagerstrom, 1996; Henningfield et al., 1995). For example, cigarette smokers weigh about 5 to 10 pounds less than nonsmokers (Grunberg, 1992). Smokers who quit tend to increase their body weight by the same amount, with a small percentage of people gaining much more weight and some even losing weight. The postcessation weight gain also occurs in animals that have been given nicotine over some time and are then taken off nicotine. Through its modulation of the appetite-controlling brain hormone serotonin, nicotine may reduce appetite. Nicotine reduces the desirability of sweet-tasting foods. It can also increase the rate of food metabolism by the equivalent of about one candy bar per day (100 to 200 calories; Grunberg, 1992).

In addition, nicotine modulates mood and performance (Balfour & Fagerstrom, 1996; Henningfield et al., 1995). Similarly, nicotine may reduce anxiety and depression, although not to the extent that antidepressant medications or *anxiolytic* (anxiety-reducing) drugs reduce symptoms. Overall, nicotine-

dependent tobacco users learn that they feel discomfort when attempting abstinence from nicotine and that continued nicotine intake makes them feel better.

Summary

As shown in this chapter, nicotine produces many and diverse effects that
can add up to a powerful grip on behavior. Some of these effects might be considered beneficial if it were not for the fact that the most common forms of nicotine
are so deadly. For example, the weight-controlling, mood-modulating, and possi-
bly performance-enhancing effects of tobacco-delivered nicotine appear to rival
those of some drugs that have been approved for treating people with weight,
mood, and cognitive dysfunction problems. Of course, it is important to recognize
that nicotine has not actually been approved by the Food and Drug Administration
as a potential treatment for disorders other than tobacco dependence.

It is also possible that the cigarette, which maximizes the addictive effects of
nicotine by producing explosively high dose levels in the arterial blood stream,
also maximizes the apparently beneficial effects of nicotine. In other words, it is
possible that the beneficial effects of nicotine, like the addictive effects, are maxi-
mized by the dosing conditions unique to cigarette smoke inhalation. In that case,
the benefits are obviously not worth the 50% risk of premature death, particularly
because other safer drugs and therapies are proven to be effective in achieving the
same beneficial effects. On the other hand, it is also likely that at least part of the
apparent benefit of nicotine may be secondary to the relief of withdrawal symptoms in nicotine-dependent users (Balfour & Fagerstrom, 1996; Royal College of
Physicians, 2000).

Researchers need further time and study to determine whether or not nicotine
in safer forms of delivery (such as gum and patches) can be considered a beneficial
drug. However, as a review by Balfour and Fagerstrom (1996) suggests, many potential medical applications of nicotine go beyond the treatment of tobacco dependence. Furthermore, it is possible that variations on the nicotine molecule will
lead to new medicines that will heighten the desired beneficial effects of nicotine
while reducing the undesirable effects (e.g., Adler et al., 1998). The dawn of the
20th century witnessed the application of nicotine to explore the nervous system
(Langley, 1906). Perhaps the dawn of the 21st century will be marked by the application of nicotine to treat disorders of the nervous system. In any case, many roads
still need to be explored before we fully understand all the ways that nicotine affects the human body.

Further Reading

Benowitz, N. L. (Ed.). (1998). *Nicotine safety and toxicity.* New York: Oxford University Press.

This excellent review makes use of chapters written by leading experts on nicotine to provide guidance on the risks and benefits of nicotine-containing medicines.

Royal College of Physicians. (2000). *Nicotine addiction in Britain: A report of the tobacco advisory group of the Royal College of Physicians.* London: Royal College of Physicians of London.

This report contains an up-to-date review of the effects of nicotine on the body and how the effects compare with those of other addictive drugs.

U.S. Department of Health and Human Services. (1988). *Nicotine addiction—A report of the surgeon general.* Washington, DC: U.S. Department of Health and Human Services.

This is one of the most complete assessments of the effects of nicotine.

5

The Natural History
of a Dependence Disorder

*By inhaling, the smoker can get nicotine in his brain
more rapidly than the heroin addict can get
a "buzz" when he shoots heroin into a vein.*

—Russell and Feyerabend (1978)

About two thirds of college students have tried tobacco, but far fewer of them will use tobacco throughout their lives. What risk factors make a person susceptible to long-term smoking? And what is it about cigarettes that draws a young person toward experimentation and then moves him or her on to regular use? This chapter explores some of those forces, including cultural attitudes about smoking, biological vulnerability, and tobacco's reinforcing properties.

Picture a 12-year-old hunched over on the front steps of an apartment building and injecting a drug into a vein in her arm—a sight most people would find shocking, because of her age and because the setting is so public. Picture now a similar adolescent taking a drag on a cigarette. The sight of a young person smoking is so common that many people would not find it surprising, and many would be unlikely to give it a second thought or to wonder why she is smoking. As a whole, society seems to have little understanding of why people use drugs, including the drug nicotine.

Why do most people smoke? Most smokers use cigarettes to experience the effects of nicotine on the central nervous system (United States Department of Health and Human Services [USDHHS], 1988; Royal College of Physicians [RCP], 2000). They also smoke because, through repeated exposure to tobacco, they have come to find smoking to be highly reinforcing. Most people develop an addiction to nicotine within days, weeks, or months of using tobacco on a regular basis. Complex biobehavioral factors underlie this addiction. Nicotine is not the only factor, but it is the critical factor. A tobacco product that failed to deliver nicotine probably would be less of a commercial success, even if it had a potent and seductive marketing campaign. Nonetheless, many of the factors that lead people to take up smoking are the same influences that drive other consumer purchases.

The title of this chapter comes from an essay by one of the most influential researchers on nicotine and tobacco, Michael Russell (1971). The title was also used for a chapter in a recent British RCP (2000) report, *Nicotine Addiction in Britain*. It is fitting to acknowledge Russell's approach to this topic, because Russell, a research psychiatrist, identifies recruitment to cigarette use as a biobehavioral process that is critically influenced by the effects of nicotine. Psychosocial factors, such as children attempting to act grown-up or being rebellious, are reasons why people initially try smoking; but if cigarettes failed to deliver nicotine to the brain, few people would be likely to use them compulsively.

■ Before the First Cigarette

Aspects of a culture can encourage or discourage smoking. Research shows that children have distinct ideas about the good things that smoking might do for them (Lloyd & Lucas, 1998; Lynch & Bonnie, 1994). Surveys of adolescents in California found that two thirds believed that smoking helps people socialize, relax, and lose weight (Pierce et al., 1993). Advertising and promotions can make smoking seem fashionable and desirable. One analysis proposes that key advertising themes that influence children include the following (Lynch & Bonnie, 1994, p. 82):

- Tobacco is a rite of passage to adulthood.
- Successful, attractive people use tobacco.
- Tobacco use is normal.
- Tobacco is safe and healthful.
- Tobacco use is relaxing in social situations.

These advertising themes, which arise in response to analyses of factors that motivate people to smoke, appeal to people's needs and desires. Many attribute an increase in youth smoking over the last two decades to an upsurge in the distribution of tobacco industry promotional items and sponsorships. The promotional expenditure budget for U.S. tobacco companies climbed from about $1 billion in the mid-1980s to about $6 billion by the early 1990s, according to Federal Trade Commission data (FTC, 1999a). Promotional items include displays, promotional allowances, samples, direct mail, entertainment sponsorships, endorsements, and testimonials. Promotional efforts tracked by the FTC did not overtly include the form of advertising called *product placement,* which is a common marketing technique of paying film and television producers to display products prominently on screen (Glantz, Slade, Bero, Hanauer, & Barnes, 1996, pp. 364-374). A product placement contract could involve a tobacco company paying a filmmaker to have a specific character in a film smoke a cigar for a certain length of time in certain scenes, shot from certain angles to maximize product exposure. These invisible, unregulated advertisements generally go unnoticed by a public engrossed in the plot of a film. Thus, at a time when tobacco could not be advertised legally on television or radio, it was marketed widely through an unregulated, nonadvertisement mechanism.

At the same time that promotional budgets soared, youth tobacco smoking increased. Even though health awareness was reflected in declining smoking rates among adults, particularly more educated adults, youth smoking rates climbed. In addition, the use of smokeless tobacco products became more common, especially among young men. Another co-occurrence of the promotion and increased use of a product was the rise of cigar use in the 1990s, which closely corresponded to product placement of cigars in films and television programs and was reinforced by the launch of mass-market publications lauding cigars (FTC, 1999b; National Cancer Institute, 1998).

No smoker is likely to claim that he or she started using tobacco because the Federal Drug Administration (FDA) did not regulate it, or because the government had failed to levy a sufficiently stiff tax on a tobacco product, or because a tobacco company logo was painted on the side of a winning race car. Similarly, a young smoker would not be likely to attribute his or her smoking to the fact that a local convenience store routinely sold tobacco to teenagers or to the fact that the opening credits of a popular television series featured the male star smoking a cigar. Nonetheless, statistics indicate that these are exactly the influences that increase or decrease tobacco initiation and use, particularly among the young. Individuals, however, vary considerably in their emotional state, their level of adjustment, and their coping skills. All of these conditions can interact to make a young person more or less likely to be influenced by a culture that promotes tobacco and thus to adopt a regular habit of using cigarettes.

In summary, among the many factors influencing overall smoking initiation and use rates are the following:

- Attachment of tobacco company identity to popular events and causes
- Availability of tobacco
- Economic conditions
- Government regulation of tobacco products
- Laws limiting youth access
- Marketing strategies, including role models and media depictions of tobacco use
- Tobacco taxes

Table 5.1 outlines the proposed stages of recruitment to cigarette smoking. Biological and psychosocial factors that support or discourage cigarette use are indicated.

A belief that smoking is a normal, common behavior is a dominant factor leading to the initiation of smoking (Lynch & Bonnie, 1994; Sussman et al., 1988). Seeing others smoke can make smoking appear to be a reasonable behavior. Peer pressure is one reason for trying and continuing to smoke cigarettes. In addition, seeing attractive individuals smoke can make smoking seem appealing. Children are often mistaken about how many people actually smoke.

Depictions of tobacco use in television and movies can provide subtle yet powerful exposure to tobacco messages. A sampling of 3 weeks of prime-time television in fall 1992 indicated that 1 in 4 programs contained at least one "tobacco event," which included antismoking messages. About one tobacco event occurred per hour of television, with dramas containing more tobacco events than comedies. More than 90% of tobacco events depicted tobacco positively, with men performing 3 times as many smoking acts as women. Smokers were depicted as being middle-class or wealthy, with two thirds in professional or techni-

TABLE 5.1 Stages in Childhood/Adolescent Development of Cigarette Use, Along With Sample Psychosocial/Behavioral and Biological Factors For and Against Progression to Cigarette Addiction

Stages	Psychosocial/Behavioral Factors		Biological Factors	
	Factors Supporting Dependence	*Factors Not Supporting Dependence*	*Factors Supporting Dependence*	*Factors Not Supporting Dependence*
Preparing	Family, peer attitudes about smoking; curiosity, rebelliousness, social confidence; advertising, movie placements	Family, peer attitudes and examples of not smoking; perception of health risks; school, community attitudes	Undetermined	Undetermined
Trying (Using at Least One Cigarette)	Same as Preparing; availability of cigarettes; perception that smoking is common	Same as Preparing; lack of access to cigarettes or other tobacco	Pleasant, strong reactions to inhaled smoke	Unpleasant sensory or central nervous system effects
Experimenting (Using Less Than Weekly)	Same as Trying; psychosocial rewards; additional social situations promoting smoking; low cigarette-refusal skills	Same as Trying; cost of cigarettes	Same as Trying	Same as Trying
Regular Use (Smoking Weekly to Daily)	Same as Experimenting; few smoking restrictions; perception of liking cigarettes and being a smoker; use of alcohol and other psychoactive substances	Same as Experimenting	Same as Experimenting; more experience controlling smoke dose, which improves biological effect; use of alcohol and other psychoactive substances	Same as Experimenting; adverse effects on respiratory system, e.g., asthma, feeling winded; withdrawal effects

cal occupations. Smokers were more often good guys than bad guys (Hazan & Glantz, 1995).

Popular feature films are also rife with tobacco events. More than one third of film segments examined from 62 randomly selected films had a reference to tobacco (Hazan, Lipton, & Glantz, 1994). Tobacco use was not portrayed as changing much over the 30 years depicted in the films. Although major characters in later films were less likely to be smokers than were characters in earlier films, smoking depicted among female and African-American characters increased. Even more dramatic, however, was the rise in depicting young persons as smokers; tobacco events among smokers aged 18 to 29 more than doubled. And even though smoking among elite characters decreased across the decades, smoking by elite characters was 3 times as prevalent as it was in the population.

Contributing to these perceptions may have been the depiction of tobacco characters in the *Weekly Reader,* a staple publication in elementary-school education (Balbach & Glantz, 1995). In 1992, Joe Camel himself was pictured in full color on the cover of the sixth-grade edition of the grade-school periodical—one of eight times the character appeared in it. Although this practice has been discontinued and Joe Camel has been consigned to the pages of tobacco history, the children who saw these articles and pictures as children are young adults at this writing and remain in a high-risk time period for initiating and maintaining tobacco use.

The 1998 agreements between the U.S. states and the tobacco industry limited advertising that would influence children to experiment with tobacco. Evidence establishing the effectiveness of tobacco advertising in influencing young persons to use tobacco is compelling (Bauer, Johnson, Hopkins, & Brooks, 2000). Researcher Paul M. Fischer and his colleagues (1991) reported that some 30% of 3-year-olds could identify Joe Camel. Research by John Pierce and his colleagues (1998) indicated that among adolescents, Joe Camel advertisements were the most popular. Young persons who had a favorite advertisement were the most likely to be smokers several years later. Other researchers reported that brands of cigarettes most frequently smoked by youth were most likely to be advertised in magazines with a higher percentage of young readers (King, Siegal, Celebucki, & Connolly, 1998).

Although much remains to be learned about the course of the development of nicotine dependence, a clear picture has emerged from scientific studies (Henningfield, Michaelides, & Sussman, 2000). Most people who use tobacco start in adolescence. Rigotti, Lee, and Wechsler (2000) report that tobacco use is common among college students, based on a survey of 119 four-year colleges. A total of

38% of college men and 30% of college women reported currently using tobacco; 53% of men and 41% of women had used tobacco within the previous year. Cigarettes were the most common form of tobacco used, although 16% of men and 4% of women also reported currently using cigars. Some 9% of men and less than 1% of women used smokeless tobacco. Overall, 68% of men and 57% of women (a combined total of 61%) reported ever using tobacco. Interestingly, 51% of those who had used tobacco in the previous year had used more than one tobacco product during that time, with 36% using two tobacco products and 14% using three tobacco products. Cigarettes and cigars were the most common combination of tobacco products. The median age at which these tobacco users had first tried cigarettes was 14 for both sexes.

These numbers correspond to other reports of tobacco initiation and regular use among young persons. By age 18, nearly two thirds of all youth in the United States have tried at least one cigarette (Centers for Disease Control and Prevention [CDC], 1998a). The number of persons younger than 18 who have smoked a cigarette has climbed steadily since the late 1980s. For example, in 1995, nearly 2.4 million young persons in the United States became smokers. Of these, about 1.17 million became daily smokers. This represents 75% of all new smokers in the United States for that year.

A major question is this: Among those who try cigarettes, who will go on to use tobacco on a regular basis? Recent advances in behavioral genetics have begun to detect complex interactions between environmental and biological/genetic factors that influence tobacco use. A study of the onset of alcohol drinking and tobacco smoking among twins found that shared environmental factors accounted for similarities in the age of first use of both substances. However, the time from first use to the development of regular patterns of use was influenced more by genetics than by environment. The authors concluded that their data supported other scientific literature indicating that the initiation of substance use is influenced largely by environmental factors rather than by genetics (Stallings, Hewitt, Beresford, Health, & Eaves, 1999). A study of female twins also found separate factors influencing initiation of smoking and nicotine dependence; although the etiological factors leading to both initiation and dependence overlapped, they were not identical (Kendler et al., 1999). A twin study comparing adolescents with young adults determined that the initiation of smoking in adolescents (aged 12-16) was influenced by environmental factors, although tobacco use in young adults (ages 17-25) was associated with genetic risk factors (Koopmans, van Doornen, & Boomsma, 1997). These and other studies point to the importance of psychosocial factors in smoking initiation by young persons.

Other researchers have attempted to predict who will become a smoker. Review articles report that family approval, peer use, school influences, and availability all predict later smoking (Biglan, Duncan, Ary, & Smolkowski, 1995; CDC, 1996a, 1996b, 1996c; USDHHS, 1994). In general, adolescents are more likely to take up smoking if other family members smoke. Having a best friend who smokes is also a statistical predictor of trying cigarettes; having a majority of friends who smoke predicts smoking more than one cigarette (Leventhal, Glynn, & Fleming, 1987).

▨ Trying the First Cigarette

With the first inhaled cigarette, biological elements are important, even though psychosocial factors can prevent a person from ever trying even one cigarette. One large study attempted to predict which British schoolchildren would become smokers (Bynner, 1969). The strongest predictors of recruitment to smoking were the following:

- ▨ Low fear of getting cancer
- ▨ Wanting to be grown-up
- ▨ Parental permissiveness
- ▨ The number of friends who smoked

Of those who had elevated scores on these factors, 7 of 10 became smokers. In contrast, those with low scores smoked no cigarettes. This pattern indicates that psychosocial factors such as those above can help determine who smokes as well as who does not smoke. Never-smokers are a group for whom biological influences, such as genetically based pharmacological reactions to inhaled cigarette smoke (Kozlowski, 1991), are not important influences, because the vulnerability is never tapped.

Trying cigarettes engages a complex biobehavioral process. A person who initiates tobacco use largely for psychosocial reasons may then be biologically influenced to smoke on a regular basis (Kozlowski & Herman, 1984). Negative reactions to the first exposure to tobacco can be a deterrent to later tobacco use (Kozlowski & Harford, 1976; Silverstein, Feld, & Kozlowski, 1980; Silverstein, Kelly, Swan, & Kozlowski, 1982). On the other hand, a strong negative reaction to the first cigarette may actually promote later tobacco use among some individuals (Pomerleau, Collins, Shiffman, & Pomerleau, 1993).

▦ Experimentation and Regular Use

British researcher Michael Russell (1990) wrote of what he called "the nicotine addiction trap," in which those who smoked as few as four cigarettes had a statistically greater likelihood of becoming smokers for life. His findings underscore the problem that the public—particularly the young public—is not given much scientifically accurate information about the strength of nicotine addiction and the symptoms of nicotine dependence. Many daily smokers believe that they will not be smoking in 5 years, although about 75% of this group will still be smoking 5 to 6 years later (CDC, 2000a). Schoolgirls aged 11 to 14 in England who smoked cigarettes were found to have nicotine exposure similar to that of adult smokers (McNeill, Jarvis, Stapleton, West, & Bryant, 1989), and early in their tobacco use they reported withdrawal symptoms occurring when they could not smoke (McNeill, West, Jarvis, Jackson, & Bryant, 1986).

Several life circumstances can interrupt this progression, however. Wakefield et al. (2000) indicated that smoking restrictions at home appear to slow the movement toward regular smoking and lower the prevalence of tobacco use. Restrictions in public places had a similar effect, although school-based smoking bans were effective only to the degree that adolescents believed that their fellow students were following the rules and that the rules were being enforced. Another recent study (Farkas, Gilpin, White, & Pierce, 2000) also found that adolescents living in smoke-free households were significantly less likely to be smokers and were almost twice as likely to have quit smoking than adolescents living in homes with no smoking restrictions. In addition, interventions such as community and statewide antitobacco programs appear to influence young persons to avoid experimentation, to not begin smoking on a regular basis, and to quit (Bauer, Johnson, Hopkins, & Brooks, 2000; state and local legislative actions designed to reduce tobacco use are detailed in a monograph, National Cancer Institute, 2000).

Most persons—and, in fact, many other mammals—are susceptible to developing an addiction to nicotine (e.g., Corrigall, 1999). In addition to a physical dependence on nicotine, humans' innate ability to learn through reinforcement creates an essential vulnerability to drug addiction. From an evolutionary perspective, reinforcement is vital to survival, in that it leads an organism to eat foods, reproduce, and experience beneficial and pleasurable activities. However, humans evolved to their present level many centuries before tobacco and other substances of abuse were employed.

Nicotine can be viewed as a *primary* or *direct reinforcer.* Because of its biological actions on the body, nicotine produces effects perceived as rewarding or beneficial. This causes humans and other animals to work to obtain nicotine (Corrigall & Coen, 1989). In other words, nicotine is a *positive reinforcer* of behavior. Another example of positive reinforcement would involve training a dog to sit on command by reinforcing its sitting behavior with dog biscuits. Some substances, such as nicotine, activate neuronal circuitry that is also activated by other primary sources of pleasure and emotion (e.g., see Corrigall, Franklin, Coen, & Clarke, 1992). Over time, and with repeated nicotine exposure, various behavioral and physiological processes establish the tobacco product as a powerful reinforcer. Separate from nicotine's addictive qualities, nicotine and tobacco's actions as reinforcers make breaking tobacco-related behaviors difficult.

The reinforcing effects of tobacco can be considered as both psychological and physiological, but these distinctions become blurred under scrutiny. For example, the subjective effects of tobacco use (e.g., the physical pleasure of smoking) can be closely related to the amount of nicotine used, the rapidity of use, and the time since the last dose; conversely, the severity of withdrawal symptoms can be modulated by the environmental setting (Henningfield, Schuh, & Heishman, 1995; Hurt & Robertson, 1988).

Through a process known as *conditioning,* sensory stimuli associated with the effects of nicotine can also become powerfully reinforcing. These include the sight, feel, and taste of cigarettes, as well as the effects of various smoke constituents, including nicotine, on the mouth, nose, throat, and lungs. Environmental stimuli such as being with friends who smoke, hearing a telephone ring, seeing a tobacco advertisement, or drinking a cup of coffee eventually signal a desire to smoke. This conditioned response is so strong that some smokers feel compelled to smoke whenever they answer the telephone or start the car. For these smokers, such stimuli do more than set the occasion; they elicit powerful urges that occur throughout the day, even in a smoker who already has been using tobacco throughout the day. Such effects of environmental stimuli also have been documented as important factors in addictions to heroin, cocaine, and alcohol (USDHHS, 1988).

Nicotine itself directly reinforces the behavior of smoking tobacco. Because direct reinforcement occurs repeatedly for smokers, the reinforced behaviors involved in seeking, lighting, and smoking cigarettes become entrenched. These behaviors become conditioned both through positive and negative reinforcement processes. Specifically, the stimulation of nicotine receptors in the brain and the activation of the dopaminergic reward system mediate the ability of nicotine to produce pleasurable effects and positive reinforcement (Corrigall, 1999). It is plausible that inhaling cigarette smoke optimizes these reinforcing effects because the nicotine in cigarette smoke rapidly affects the brain's nicotinic receptors. Yet it is unlikely that each separate puff has a dramatic effect on the brain, in part because an acute tolerance can develop after the first few puffs or first few cigarettes of the day (Kozlowski, 1982). In addition, nicotine administration also provides relief from the symptoms of withdrawal, which begin to emerge within a few hours of abstinence. Nicotine replacement medications, such as the gum or the patch, lessen withdrawal symptoms but with fewer pleasurable sensations than are provided by smoke inhalation (Henningfield, 1995). Thus, with nicotine replacement medications, the cigarette smoker may obtain the nicotine he or she needs to avoid withdrawal, but the smoker will have few of the pleasurable sensations produced by tobacco use.

Summary

Clearly, not everyone who first experiments with tobacco progresses to regular and even lifetime use. However, cigarettes are both addictive and reinforcing. The environmental susceptibility that many young persons experience can lead to their becoming addicted to nicotine through biological means that may be at least partially genetically influenced. Tobacco's reinforcing traits can make quitting particularly difficult, because the smoker must break not only the addiction to nicotine but also the highly reinforced behaviors associated with smoking.

Further Reading

Lynch, B. S., & Bonnie, R. J. (Eds.). (1994). *Growing up tobacco free: Preventing nicotine addiction in children and youths.* Washington, DC: Institute of Medicine, National Academy Press

This provides a thorough review of issues related to smoking and youth.

Russell, M. A. H. (1971). Cigarette smoking: Natural history of a dependence disorder. *British Journal of Medical Psychology, 44,* 1-16.

This classic work helped to establish an influential framework for research on this topic. Note how the principles identified in 1971 still apply in 2001.

U.S. Department of Health and Human Services. (1994). *Preventing tobacco use among young people: A report of the surgeon general.* Washington, DC: U.S. Department of Health and Human Services, Public Health Service, Centers for Disease Control and Prevention, National Center for Chronic Disease Prevention and Health Promotion, Office of Smoking and Health.

This extensive review provides an excellent resource for learning more about research and public health issues related to the prevention of youth smoking.

6

Tobacco Use as Nicotine Addiction

I'd rather give up heroin than smokes.

—Anonymous client,
Addiction Research
Foundation of Ontario, 1988

The terms *addicts* and *addiction* have a secure place in the popular culture. When we talk of television junkies, jogging nuts, drug addicts, compulsive gamblers, chocoholics, obsessive Net surfers, or alcoholics, we make some use of the concept of addiction. The term *addiction* has never applied just to drug use. In fact, although the *Oxford English Dictionary* (Murray, Bradley, Craigre, & Onions, 1933) records that the label was applied to wine and tobacco consumption in the 18th century, it also cites the use of the terms *addicted* and *addiction* to describe the compulsion to dance, read, obtain money, and preserve virginity. Thus, for centuries, the focus of the concept of addiction has been on behavior, specifically, on behavior that appears excessive or compulsive and that appears to be ruled by some desire, force, or drive outside the individual's full control.

In the 20th century, however, considerable baggage has been added to the term *addiction* (Jaffe, 1990). Most influential has been the popular image of the criminal heroin addict: an immoral person who would sell his mother's wheelchair, rob a convenience store, or murder a passerby to get money for a drug "fix." This heroin addict is viewed as a wretched victim of the morally decaying effects of the drug and who has no control over the physical symptoms that occur when he or she runs out of drugs. Such florid popular images of so-called hard drug addicts understandably make some people doubt that nicotine users ever deserve to be considered addicted.

In contrast to this picture, many families have an Uncle Charlie or Aunt Ruth who smoked for years but who one day with no special medical assistance threw away his or her cigarettes and never smoked again. It is troubling to picture Uncle Charlie or Aunt Ruth as having been addicts of the sort described above.

Popular images of heroin addiction have led to the widespread myth that "once an addict, always an addict" (Johnston, 1977). Careful research has shown that this myth does not apply even to heroin addicts (Robins, 1975, 1993). Many individuals have beaten their addictions to both cigarettes and heroin. *Inability* to stop using a drug is not a defining characteristic of a drug addiction, although *difficulty* in stopping use is (e.g., Kalant, Clarke, Corrigall, Ferrence, & Kozlowski, 1989).

Although tobacco was often included among addictions in common parlance, formal categorization of tobacco as addicting by the U.S. surgeon general is more recent. In fact, cigarette smoking was considered for potential categorization as a form of drug addiction in the landmark 1964 U.S. surgeon general's report, which found that smoking was a cause of lung cancer. That report did recognize that smoking could be habitual and difficult to stop and that nicotine was an important chemical factor but concluded that smoking was not appropriately considered a form of drug addiction (U.S. Department of Health, Education, and Welfare, 1964). It was not until the 1986 surgeon general's report in which the potential addicting effects of smokeless tobacco were evaluated that the surgeon general came to the firm conclusion that nicotine in smokeless tobacco was addictive (U.S. Department of Health and Human Services, 1986). The topic was much more thoroughly evaluated in the 1988 surgeon general's report, which concluded that nicotine met all the criteria for classification as an addictive drug and that nicotine-delivering tobacco products were appropriately regarded as addicting (USDHHS, 1988).

What led to this change in conclusion by U.S. surgeons general from 1964 to the 1980s? Did the definition change or were new discoveries about nicotine and tobacco made? What are the clinical signs and symptoms of tobacco use that warrant the label of addiction? Does the addiction involve a simple physical dependence on the drug nicotine, or is it more complex than that? How does nicotine compare with other addictive drugs in its addictive effects?

▨ Biobehavioral Framework for the Study of Addiction

Knowing what a drug does to the brain and the rest of the body is important, but it does not fully explain the addictive nature of a drug. The chemical structure of a drug is only one factor in determining how society or science views a drug. Psychosocial and cultural reactions to the drug can also influence drug use. A drug that produces addiction in a high percentage of its users might be thought to be more addictive than a drug that produces addiction in a small percentage of its users. The pharmacological actions of this more addictive drug might also be assumed to cause more addiction than does the less addictive drug. However, it is not enough to understand the pharmacological actions of the drug.

The following example shows the need for a biobehavioral framework. Consider the question of what proportion of alcohol users are alcohol addicts. In a "dry" (alcohol-forbidding) county in the southern United States, where any alcohol purchase is illegal, we see very little alcohol use overall but a very high percentage of alcohol addiction in those who do use alcohol. The legal restrictions and other cultural influences discourage alcohol use to the extent that all those who might otherwise use alcohol occasionally or socially do not use it at all. Those who do use alcohol are those who find it hard not to use alcohol excessively. In contrast, a "wet" (alcohol-allowing) county nearby would have more widespread alcohol use, with many persons using at least a little alcohol and a relatively small percentage of users showing alcohol addiction. This comparison of "wet" and "dry" counties (Cahalan & Room, 1974) illustrates how psychosocial and behavioral factors interact with pharmacological factors to influence what addictive drug use looks like in a specific place and time. Judging the addictiveness of a drug on the basis of the percentage of addicted users of the drug can lead to inconsistent findings, depending on the context being studied.

Drug dependence depends on more than just the chemical properties of the drug. The percentage of persons who are able to stop using drugs varies widely from context to context. For example, heroin use was common among U.S. soldiers participating in the Vietnam War in the 1960s and 1970s. After returning to the United States, more than 80% of these veterans returned to some level of heroin use. However, within 3 years, more than 90% of these users were abstinent from heroin and similar drugs. The classic studies of these drug users by Lee Robins (Robins, 1993) has had profound implications for our understanding of drug addiction. They showed that, even for heroin, it was not true that "once an addict, always an addict." Changes in the environment can lead to abstinence even when the most powerfully addictive drugs are involved.

The persistence and course of drug addiction involve more than the chemically mediated effects of an addictive substance. A psychoactive drug is an important determinant of the addictive behavior, but this does not imply that other environmental factors are not important modulators of addiction. For example, individuals often acquire a strong preference for a particular method of ingesting their addictive drug of choice. Some prefer smoking, some prefer injecting drugs, and some would rather swallow their favored drug. Factors such as price also are strong determinants of consumption. Psychosocial and situational pressures can drive an individual's nicotine intake up or down. Biologically influenced boundaries can determine when an addict's nicotine use becomes too little or too much: the lower boundary can result from withdrawal discomfort; the upper boundary can result from the acute toxic effects of smoking (Benowitz, Jacob, Kozlowski, & Yu, 1986; Kozlowski & Herman, 1984). Both animals and humans tend to consume more of a drug when it is low in cost or effort to obtain and less as the price rises. Both animals and humans tend to demonstrate more extreme addictive behavior in response to drugs and drug dosage forms that provide rapid effects than to those that have a slower onset.

Historically, tobacco addiction has been most obvious when psychosocial and situational factors reveal what some individuals will do to obtain tobacco. When the health risks of cigarette smoking were not yet clear and cigarettes were readily available, as was true in the early 20th century in the United States, cigarette smoking appeared to be a bad habit rather than a true drug addiction. On the other hand, the images of smokers selling food rations for tobacco and scrounging for cigarette butts in the streets, as was true in Germany at the end of World War II (see Brecher, 1972), indicate the strength of tobacco addiction. Decades of detailed research and the development of new research tools (e.g., ways to measure nicotine levels in the blood and animal models to assess the behavioral effects of nicotine) were needed to establish that *tobacco* addiction was *nicotine* addiction.

The Concepts of Addiction and Dependence

To understand drug addiction, it is important to separate popular, fictional accounts of addiction from accounts provided by scientific study. In the scientific literature, the terms *drug addiction* and *drug dependence* have specific meanings. They refer to the repeated, and frequently harmful, use of a drug that affects the brain in a way that sustains drug seeking—drug use that is difficult for the user to stop, despite many reasons and multiple attempts to do so. This does not mean that terminating drug use is impossible or even difficult for all drug users. Indeed, as observed earlier, more than 90% of military personnel who had been using heroin and heroin-like drugs in Vietnam ceased their use within a few years of their return to the United States—many without formal treatment (Robins, 1993; USDHHS, 1988). Additional criteria are discussed later in this chapter.

The concept of *control* is imbedded in addiction theory. Drug addiction involves an interaction between chemistry, behavior, and physiology that leads to the compulsive behavior whereby the drug itself acquires substantial control over the individual. Although people often consider drug addiction to involve behavior that is out of control, in reality the behavior of the individual is under exquisite control—control by the drug. However, control is not exerted solely by the drug. For example, studies at the Johns Hopkins and Harvard medical schools in the 1970s showed that seemingly out-of-control alcoholic research volunteers regulated their alcohol intake in accordance with social factors, such as the opportunity to drink with others, and with behavioral factors, such as the cost per drink (Griffiths, Bigelow, & Henningfield, 1980). Participants preferred to delay drinking if it provided a later opportunity to drink with others, and they drank less when the price was increased. Thus, rather than simply being captives of the chemical actions of alcohol, the alcoholics could alter their behavior by the same kinds of factors that determine other sorts of behaviors.

The 1964 report to the surgeon general concluded that the use of tobacco was "reinforced and perpetuated by the pharmacological actions of nicotine on the central nervous system" (USDHEW, 1964, p. 354). The report further concluded that "nicotine-free tobacco or plant materials do not satisfy the needs of those who acquire the tobacco habit" (p. 354). Clearly, that report implied that nicotine was a critical factor in controlling the behavior of the tobacco user. However, the report categorized nicotine as *habituating* rather than *addicting,* according to criteria adapted from a 1957 expert committee of the World Health Organization (World Health Organization [WHO], 1957; U. S. Department of Health Education and Welfare, 1964; USDHHS, 1988). Part of the distinction between habituating and addicting was that addicting drugs were believed to exert stronger control over users than habituating drugs. And as shown in the earlier example of wet and dry counties, the context can have a large effect on the apparent strength of the control exerted by a drug.

■ Criteria for Addiction

The 1957 WHO criteria were developed to identify potentially dangerous drugs that should be controlled through regulation and trade restriction to protect the public. The most dangerous were those meeting criteria for producing drug addiction; those warranting less control were those meeting criteria for drug habituation. Habituating drugs were thought to be capable of sustaining repeated consumption due to some degree of psychological dependence that created a desire (but not a compulsion) to use the drug. Such drugs were thought to exert detrimental effects primarily on the individual. Addicting drugs were believed to produce a compulsion to use as well as psychological dependence, physical dependence, an escalation in use over time, and detrimental effects on society as well as on the individual.

Drugs such as morphine and pentobarbital were considered addicting by the 1957 WHO criteria. Amphetamine was considered habituating. Cocaine was treated as though it were an addictive drug even though it was anomalous in that it did not clearly meet the criteria for dose escalation, physical dependence, and compulsion to use (Gold, 1993). Alcohol was generally considered addictive even though most users of alcohol displayed few classic signs of addiction. Alcoholic beverages were excluded from regulation by the WHO. Tobacco was not even considered in written reports by the expert committees of the WHO, which addressed psychoactive and addicting drugs.

An additional consideration in the identification of addicting drugs was that the process of addiction was widely thought to reflect serious psychological weakness and personality disorder on the part of the addicted person. This was thought to explain why not all who used an addictive drug became addicted. It also gave comfort to regular users of tobacco that surely they could not be addicted. Interestingly, the key drug addiction expert on the 1964 advisory committee to the surgeon general was himself a cigarette smoker considered acceptable as a committee member by the tobacco industry (Jarvik, 1995).

Nonetheless, the same WHO committee that distinguished between addicting and habituating drugs in the 1950s dropped the distinction in 1964, recognizing that the distinction was unclear (WHO, 1964; USDHHS, 1988). They recognized that cocaine merited strong regulatory controls even though it did not clearly appear to meet criteria as an addicting drug. The common feature across the drugs of concern was that they produced psychological ("psychic") dependence and often, but not always, tolerance and physical dependence. Thus, the two terms addicting and habituating were replaced by the single term *dependence*. *Dependence* was also considered to be a more neutral scientific term, devoid of the adverse social and moral connotations of *addiction*. This advance by WHO was apparently too late for consideration by the surgeon general's committee, which issued its report on nicotine in the same year.

Although the term *dependence* is technically useful, nonexperts tend to view dependence as something less than addiction even though that was never the intent of the WHO. Organizations and individuals such as the National Institute on Drug Abuse, the American Society of Addiction Medicine, the Royal Society of Canada, the Royal College of Physicians in the United Kingdom, and the U.S. surgeon general continue to prefer *addiction* in many communications, especially with the general public (Food and Drug Administration, 1996).

▉ Evidence and Theory Progress Hand-in-Hand

Even if the criteria for dependence had not changed in 1964, the patterns of tobacco use and the pharmacological effects of nicotine discovered in the 1970s and 1980s would have led to nicotine's being categorized as addicting. In the early 1960s, unequivocal evidence that the compulsion to use tobacco could equal that of morphine did not exist. That evidence was gathered in 1988. At the time of the 1964 report, relatively little research existed on cigarette smoking as an addiction. The evidence for physical dependence and withdrawal was preliminary before 1980. Moreover, the evidence that nicotine could produce psychologically reinforcing effects in humans and animals was weak until the 1980s. Major discoveries of the late 1970s and 1980s included the following findings:

■ Compulsion to self-administer tobacco products despite potential harm can be as strong as that for morphine.

- Repeated use produces physical dependence.
- Use escalates considerably from initial levels in most people.
- Nontobacco forms of nicotine can substitute for the reinforcing effects of tobacco in animals and humans.
- Society and nonusers of tobacco often suffer adverse consequences of smoking.
- High doses of nicotine can intoxicate, even though this rarely occurs among practiced tobacco users (Royal College of Physicians, 2000; USDHHS, 1988).

Concepts of addiction did evolve, but so did the progress of scientific discovery that confirmed that by either set of nomenclature, nicotine was a powerful drug that could lead humans to use tobacco products despite the risk of harm to themselves and others. In 1982, National Institute on Drug Abuse Director Dr. William Pollin testified before the U.S. Congress that nicotine met all criteria for a dependence-producing drug, on par with morphine and cocaine (USDHHS, 1984).

Nicotine's addictive properties were reviewed in a section of the 1986 surgeon general's report that concluded that smokeless tobacco was addictive and harmful (USDHHS, 1986). That report made it clear that numerous discoveries over the preceding decade confirming the addictive effects of nicotine warranted a full report focusing on addiction. This led to the development of the surgeon general's 1988 report, *Nicotine Addiction,* under the leadership of Dr. C. Everett Koop (USDHHS, 1988). The 1988 report found that by all of the criteria in Table 6.1, nicotine was appropriately categorized as an addictive or dependence-producing drug.

The three major conclusions of the 1988 report were:

1. Cigarettes and other forms of tobacco are addicting.
2. Nicotine is the drug in tobacco that causes addiction.
3. The pharmacological and behavioral processes that determine tobacco addiction are similar to those that determine addiction to drugs such as heroin and cocaine.

Other organizations and committees around the world confirmed these conclusions of the surgeon general (Food and Drug Administration, 1996; Royal College of Physicians, 2000). On the basis of these conclusions, as well as on the evidence that the tobacco industry willfully and intentionally manufactured its products to produce and sustain addiction, the FDA proposed regulating cigarettes and

TABLE 6.1 Criteria for Dependence-Producing Drugs

Primary criteria

- Highly controlled or compulsive use
- Psychoactive effects
- Drug-reinforced behavior

Additional criteria

- Addictive behavior often involves—
  Stereotypic patterns of use
  Use despite harmful effects
  Relapse following abstinence
  Recurrent drug cravings
- Dependence-producing drugs often produce—
  Tolerance
  Physical dependence
  Pleasant (euphoriant) effects

SOURCE: U.S. Department of Health and Human Services (1988).

smokeless tobacco as drugs under the auspices of the Federal Food Drug and Cosmetic Act (FDA, 1996; Kessler et al., 1996). The tobacco industry was the only major body that disputed the conclusions of the surgeon general or the FDA.

An expert committee report for the Health Protection Branch of Health and Welfare Canada (Kalant et al., 1989) offered a definition of addiction that overlaps with that used in the 1988 surgeon general's report, although it has a different emphasis:

> Drug addiction is a strongly established pattern of behaviour characterized by (1) the repeated self-administration of a drug in amounts which reliably produce reinforcing psychoactive effects, and (2) great difficulty in achieving voluntary long-term cessation of such use, even when the user is motivated to stop. (p. v)

The expert committee concurred with the U.S. surgeon general and judged that cigarette smoking can and often does meet all the criteria of this definition of drug addiction.

Clinical Features of Nicotine Dependence and Withdrawal

The most widely recognized system of diagnosing behavioral and mental disorders is that regularly issued and updated by the American Psychiatric Association (APA). Its *Diagnostic and Statistical Manual* (*DSM*) provides clinical descriptions and systems of diagnosis that are used worldwide. In 1980, the third edition of the *DSM, DSM-III,* first categorized tobacco dependence and withdrawal syndromes. When the book was revised in 1987 (*DSM-III-R*), it substituted the term *nicotine* for *tobacco,* because by that time the role of nicotine in the compulsive use of tobacco was widely recognized as being similar to the role of cocaine in coca leaf use, morphine in opium use, and ethanol in alcoholic beverage consumption.

By the 1980s, research had established that the consumption of these substances was strongly determined by the effects of a psychoactive drug. These effects included the ability of the drug to cause tolerance, sometimes to establish physiological dependence, and to serve as an effective reinforcer. Nicotine, like other addictive drugs, had been demonstrated to be capable of serving as a powerful reinforcer for humans and animals. The reinforcing effect in animals was found in tests when animals pressed a lever to produce intravenous injections of nicotine (Goldberg, Spealman, & Goldberg, 1981).

DSM-III recognition of tobacco dependence and withdrawal helped pave the way for the conclusions of the surgeon general in 1986 and 1988. Whereas the surgeon general's reports focused primarily on nicotine's pharmacological effects, the APA focused more on clinical phenomena in developing objective criteria to guide health professional in treating patients. As described in the most recent version of the *Diagnostic and Statistical Manual, DSM-IV* (APA, 1994), the hallmark of nicotine dependence is the same as that for other drug-dependence disorders and can be described in brief as a maladaptive pattern of use often accompanied by tolerance and withdrawal. These features may have escalated from early use and may persist in the face of harm and despite repeated efforts to quit (see APA, 1994, for more specific diagnostic criteria). Symptoms of nicotine withdrawal are summarized in Table 6.2. The *DSM* undoubtedly will be revised again to reflect further advances in diagnosing and treating substance dependence and other disorders.

Despite claims by the tobacco industry that diagnostic criteria for drug dependence are so broad that they include carrot consumption and television watching as dependence disorders, less than a dozen classes of psychoactive chemical are recognized by the APA and by WHO as producing dependence. Similarly, the surgeon general's criteria include only psychoactive drugs that produce reinforcement and compulsive behavior and excludes food and environmental stimuli. The drug classes or types generally recognized as dependence producing are alcohol, amphetamine, cocaine, cannabis, hallucinogens, inhalants, phencyclidine, and

TABLE 6.2 Primary Symptoms of Nicotine Withdrawal

In persons who have been using nicotine-delivering products on a daily basis for at least several weeks, cravings and the following signs may be observed:

Dysphoric or depressed mood
Insomnia
Irritability, frustration, or anger
Anxiety
Difficulty concentrating
Restlessness
Decreased heart rate
Increased appetite or weight gain

SOURCE: American Psychiatric Association (1994).

sedatives/hypnotics/anxiolytics (hypnotics are sleep producing; anxiolytics are anxiety reducing).

The medical use of certain forms of dependence-producing drugs is excluded from being considered a drug dependence *disorder*. For example, chronic use of barbiturates for treatment of epilepsy, morphine for chronic pain treatment, oral methadone to treat heroin dependence, and nicotine medications to achieve abstinence from cigarettes are not considered disorders. Methadone and nicotine medication therapies are often referred to as *replacement* therapies, because they provide at least a partial replacement of a dangerous form of a substance with a safer medication. The risk of heroin users contracting HIV or cigarette smokers developing heart disease is substantially reduced when methadone treatment or nicotine replacement therapy is administered.

■ Severity of Nicotine Addiction

How severe is nicotine addiction? During the latter half of the 19th century and the first half of the 20th century, the term *drug addiction* was most commonly used to describe the compulsive use of alcohol or morphine. The focus on such substances led to the concept that addictive drugs caused intoxication and that termination of chronic use was accompanied by severe withdrawal symptoms. Even though intoxication was not generally present in individuals who maintained themselves with stable supplies of morphine, the sleep-producing effects of morphine-like drugs and the intoxicating effects of alcohol provided a means of differentiating these drugs from amphetamine and cocaine.

As indicated by the criteria of the 1988 surgeon general's report (USDHHS, 1988), for a drug to be considered addictive, it must be psychoactive and capable of providing reinforcement for its own self-administration. Factors such as tolerance, physical dependence, and intoxication can exacerbate the severity of the clinical syndrome and complicate treatment efforts, but they are not required elements of an addiction. Drugs with a higher likelihood of producing adverse effects are generally regarded as more severe (thus warranting restrictions) than those that produce less adverse effects, with tobacco being the noteworthy exception to this trend.

If one were to compare several addictive drugs, for example, it would quickly become evident that they differ along various dimensions and that depending on which factors were in focus, one could come to different conclusions about which drugs are of greatest concern (Giovino, Henningfield, Tomar, Escobedo, & Slade, 1995; Henningfield, Schuh, & Heishman, 1995; USDHHS, 1988). For example, despite the facts that alcoholic beverages are the most widely consumed of all APA-recognized addictive drugs and produce the most pronounced intoxication and withdrawal syndromes in daily heavy users, 15% of users develop alcohol dependence in their lifetimes and less than 10% of alcohol consumers display signs of dependence or abuse. This compares with the estimates of the FDA that more than 80% of cigarette smokers show strong signs of dependence and that nearly one half of people who start smoking escalate to dependence. On the other hand, cocaine, which was not recognized by the APA as a dependence producing drug until 1987, does not produce physical dependence and withdrawal in most users but does produce self-administration in animals and euphoriant mood effects in humans more readily than most other addictive drugs. Opioid drugs range from analgesics that lead to addictive patterns of use in less than 1% of pain patients to street heroin that can lead to lifetime rates of addiction in approximately 20% of users. Daily heroin use is reliably associated with physical dependence and withdrawal, but the syndrome is more readily managed and less critical medically than severe alcohol withdrawal.

Intoxication is not among the criteria for an addictive drug, but if it were, the effect would be strongest for alcohol, with little intoxication observed for persons sustained on stable doses of opioids, cocaine, and nicotine, even though all of these drugs can produce intoxication at high dosages. Among all addictive drugs, none is associated with a 50% risk of premature mortality except nicotine. The point of the foregoing comparisons is not to conclude that any one of these drugs is more addictive than the others. They all clearly meet criteria for being categorized as dependence producing drugs, but the different drugs produce effects that vary as a function of their pharmacology, availability, and place in society. However, it does not make sense to conclude that cigarette smoking is not addictive because it does not typically produce the intoxication of alcohol or the withdrawal of heroin or the high degree of euphoria of cocaine. Nor would it make sense to conclude that these drugs are not addicting because only a minority of users escalate to addictive patterns of use.

Most addicts use more than one addictive substance (see Chapter 7). Using multiple-drug-using addicts as "experts" on addictive substances, Kozlowski, Skinner, Kent, and Pope (1989) asked them to compare cigarettes with other addictive drugs. Addictive drugs can induce strong desires or "cravings" (Kozlowski & Wilkinson, 1987). Participants were asked to compare the strongest urge they had ever had to use cigarettes with the strongest urge for the drug that had brought them to treatment (e.g., alcohol, cocaine, heroin). Of alcohol abusers, 82% said their strongest cigarette urges were at least as strong as their strongest urges for alcohol; 45% of cocaine abusers reported that their cigarette urges were at least as strong as for cocaine. Of the participants, 57% said that it would be harder to give up cigarettes than the alcohol or drug for which they were receiving treatment; another 17% said it would be equally hard to give up cigarettes.

Tobacco-delivered nicotine is highly addictive. Nearly 20 million people try to quit smoking each year in the United States, but less than 10% have long-term success (Pierce, Fiore, Novotny, Hatziandreu, & Davis, 1989; USDHHS, 1990). Even among persons who have lost a lung or undergone major cardiovascular surgery, only about 50% maintain abstinence for more than a few weeks (USDHHS, 1988; West & Evans, 1986). Smokers tend to consider themselves addicted. In a 1999 Gallup Poll, 79% of current smokers reported that they considered themselves addicted to cigarettes (Moore, 1999). These findings are consistent with those of the 1985 National Household Survey on Drug Abuse, which showed that 84% of 12- to 17-year-old persons who smoked a pack or more of cigarettes per day felt that they "needed" or were "dependent" on cigarettes (Henningfield, Clayton, & Pollin, 1990). The data show that 12- to 17-year-olds develop tolerance, dependence, needs, graduated usage, and inability to abstain from nicotine, indicating that the addictive processes are fundamentally the same as those studied in adults (Henningfield, Clayton, & Pollin, 1990; USDHHS, 1988).

Several studies have found nicotine to be as addicting as heroin, cocaine, or alcohol (Henningfield, Clayton, & Pollin, 1990; Henningfield, Cohen, & Slade, 1991; Kozlowski et al., 1993). In fact, the probability of becoming addicted to nicotine following any exposure is much higher than that for these other substances. This was illustrated most clearly in a recent survey of drug use patterns. The 1990 National Household Survey (NHS) indicated that of people who had consumed alcoholic beverages in the past year, 30% had consumed at least once in the past week, and that among those who had binged (5 or more drinks in a row) in the past 30 days, 17% reported that they felt they needed to drink or were dependent (National Institute on Drug Abuse [NIDA], 1991). Of those who had used cocaine in the past year, 16% had used in the past week. Among those who had used cocaine 11 times or more in their lives, 8% felt they needed the drug or were dependent. By contrast, 38% of those who had ever smoked were smoking at the time of the survey and reported that they needed tobacco or felt dependent on tobacco at the time the survey was conducted (NIDA, 1991).

Cigarettes also are considered a substance of abuse, although the pattern of occasional or low-level use that characterizes most users of other addictive drugs is relatively rare for tobacco. For example, whereas only about 10 to 15% of current alcohol drinkers are considered problem drinkers, approximately 90% of cigarette smokers smoke at least five cigarettes every day (Henningfield, 1992; Henningfield et al., 1991; Kozlowski et al., 1993).

Part of the reason that only 2% to 3% of smokers successfully achieve abstinence each year (Pierce et al., 1989) may be that most people who smoke on a daily basis report that they feel dependent and have experienced withdrawal symptoms (Henningfield et al., 1990; USDHHS, 1988).

Terminology

Nomenclature has evolved as our scientific understanding of drug dependence has evolved. We now recognize that a variety of drugs can be labeled addictive and that their effects differ. These effects are described by terms including *tolerance, physical dependence, withdrawal, psychoactivity, reinforcement, abuse liability, dependence potential,* and *intoxication.* Table 6.3 provides definitions of these key terms.

Summary

Nicotine addiction has now been established as a significant, substantial drug addiction. All drug addictions are the result of complex biobehavioral processes.

TABLE 6.3 Glossary of Commonly Used Terms to Describe Addictive Drugs

Abuse: This refers to maladaptive use of a substance that may or may not produce dependence. Thus, maintaining dependence by medically supervised self-administration of methadone and transdermal nicotine is not considered abuse, even though certain effects of the substances they have replaced (i.e., street heroin and cigarettes, respectively) could be considered abuse.

Abuse liability: A drug meets criteria for abuse liability if it produces effects mediated by the brain that are sufficient to lead a substantial proportion of people and animals to repeatedly self-administer the drug. Abuse liability is confirmed by demonstrating that the drug will serve as a positive reinforcer in animals and humans and that it produces stimulus effects, which overlap with those produced by drugs of abuse, such as amphetamine and morphine.

Addiction: This is not currently used as a technical term by the American Psychiatric Association or the World Health Organization, but it is often used by these organizations and others interchangeably with *dependence* to communicate with more general audiences.

Dependence: The hallmark of dependence is that a drug with independently verifiably abuse liability is repeatedly used by an individual, frequently in spite of his or her knowledge of the potential for adverse effects.

Intoxication: Intoxication can result in disruption of behavior and cognitive function. This may be regarded as an adverse effect of a chemical that is one concern about use of the substance and may provide an incentive for some individuals to abuse the substance, but it is not an essential feature of dependence. Substances such as nicotine and amphetamine can produce intoxication; however, their use is not generally associated with intoxication, whereas alcohol and barbiturates commonly produce intoxication.

Physiological dependence: This refers to the state of behavioral and physiological adaptation to a drug such that functioning appears generally normal when the person or animal is maintained on the drug, and acute disruption occurs upon termination of drug administration. For alcohol, morphine, and nicotine, clearly observable signs of withdrawal and discomfort typically begin less than 12 hours after the last dose, and many of the signs are the opposite of those produced by acute drug administration; for example, alcohol's depressant effects on muscle tone are replaced by tremors, morphine's

(Continued)

TABLE 6.3 Continued

constipating effects are replaced by diarrhea, and nicotine's anxiolytic effects are replaced by anxiety.

Tolerance: Tolerance refers to the reduced responsiveness that occurs with repetition of dosing such that over time, increased doses are required to produce the effects initially produced by lower doses. Tolerance is rarely complete (e.g., the nausea-producing effects of nicotine and respiratory depressant effects of morphine can occur by dose increases) and varies depending on the response or symptom being measured. For example, there is little tolerance to the pupilary-constricting effects of morphine but considerable tolerance to the acute pleasurable effects produced by morphine injections and nicotine doses.

Withdrawal symptoms: These include the time-limited constellation of signs and symptoms that occurs after termination of drug administration. Their severity generally is related to the amount of drug that the person or animal had been taking on a daily basis. The severity of the symptoms generally is reduced by a gradual reduction of dosing over time.

No addicting drug gives rise to addiction in all who use the drug. Behavioral (including psychosocial and contextual) factors have dramatic effects on the nature of drug addiction. If it were not for addiction to tobacco products, the dangerous consequences of tobacco use (see Chapter 3) would likely not be a public health problem, because most smokers would not have become regular, heavy users of tobacco. Cigarette addiction can be viewed as a root cause of the death and disability arising from cigarette use.

Further Reading

American Psychiatric Association. (1994). *Diagnostic and statistical manual of mental disorders* (4th ed.). Washington, DC: American Psychiatric Association.

This text provides a detailed description of drug addictions and how they are epistemologically differentiated from compulsive behavioral disorders.

Goldstein, A. (1994). *Addiction: From biology to drug policy.* New York: Freeman.

This book by one of the leading scientists and theoreticians in addiction science provides a lucid description of the effects of a variety of addictive drugs at the receptor level to the consequences of their use at the societal level. Policy implications of basic biological findings are also discussed.

Henningfield, J. E., Schuh, L. M., & Jarvik, M. E. (1995). Pathophysiology of tobacco dependence. In F. E. Bloom & D. J. Kupfer (Eds.), *Psychopharmacology: The fourth generation of progress* (pp. 1715-1729). New York: Raven.

This chapter summarizes the biological basis for nicotine's addictive effects from the perspective that the underlying pathogenesis of nicotine addiction is at least as well understood as the pathogenesis of effects of tobacco use such as lung cancer.

Molinoff, P. B., & Ruddon, R. W. (Eds.). (1996). *Goodman & Gilman's: The pharmacological basis of therapeutics* (9th ed.). New York: McGraw-Hill.

This is the primary sourcebook for the essential pharmacology of drugs in general. Several chapters address in great detail various drugs that produce dependence, and one chapter provides an authoritative discussion of drug addiction and abuse.

Robins, L. N. (1993). Vietnam veterans' rapid recovery from heroin addiction: A fluke or normal expectation. *Addiction, 88,* 1041-1054.

This article summarizes the studies of drug use among veterans of the Vietnam War. It illustrates some of the factors that determine the course of addiction and it debunks some of the commonly held myths about drug addiction.

7

Smoking, Drinking, and Drug Taking

A Biobehavioral Syndrome

*Life is (as I have been known to say) a Three-Legged Stool,
supported by Booze, Coffee, and Smokes, which interdepend
essentially. Kick away any leg of the stool and the whole
corpus comes crashing to the kitchen floor.*

—L. Rust Hills (1993)

This chapter is about the relationship of smoking to other types of drug use. Smokers and nonsmokers differ in many ways. Smokers are more likely to have high-risk sex, less likely to wear seatbelts in cars, more likely to sleep fewer hours each night, more likely to eat fried foods, less likely to eat fruit and vegetables, more likely to drink alcohol, and more likely to use "hard" drugs (Schoenborn & Benson, 1988; Wichelow, Golding, & Treasure, 1988). In addition to these differences, there is also evidence of a kind of dose-response function: It is not just that smokers are different from nonsmokers in the above ways, but heavy smokers also experience greater effects than light smokers.

Many smokers present a syndrome—or complex pattern—of dangerous activities. How do scientists explain these clusters of activities? Is an *addictive personality* responsible for the syndrome? Is it true that smoking is a *gateway* or *stepping-stone* problem that can *cause* the smoker to be more likely to use and abuse other drugs such as alcohol, cocaine, and heroin? Or is it better to think of smoking as a risk factor for other substance use and abuse? Are those who smoke more vulnerable to using other drugs? Do genes influence multiple drug use? Biobehavioral models are needed to answer all of these questions.

■ Patterns of Tobacco Use and Other Drug Use

Overall, the patterns are clear. As a category, smokers are more likely to use other drugs than are nonsmokers. A dose-response association is present in that heavy smokers are even more likely than light smokers to use other drugs, and, if the heavy smoker uses other drugs, the level of use (e.g., drinks of alcohol per day) will also be heavier than for light smokers. This has been found to be true in many studies and countries (e.g., Cronk & Sarvela, 1997; Henningfield, Clayton, & Pollin, 1990).

Teenagers who use tobacco are 8 times more likely to use marijuana and 22 times more likely to use cocaine, according to findings from the Centers for Disease Control and Prevention (1998c). As discussed in Chapter 3, "relative risks" such as these need to be understood in light of the percentages being compared. Figure 7.1 summarizes data from interviews of 12- to 17-year-olds conducted in the United States in 1995 as part of the National Household Survey of the National Institute on Drug Abuse.

Smokers were 5 times more likely than nonsmokers to have used any alcohol in the past month (56% of smokers vs. 11 % of nonsmokers). Smokers were 9 times more likely than nonsmokers to binge drink, with 31% of smokers and only 3% of nonsmokers binge drinking in the past 30 days. (Binge drinking is defined here as drinking five or more drinks on the same occasion at least once in the past 30 days and is a small subset of overall alcohol use.) So binge drinking and "heavy drinking" (defined as drinking five or more drinks on each of five or more days) are much more likely in smokers; but overall fewer people use alcohol this much. The pattern in Figure 7.1 shows that (a) many young smokers, aged 12 to 17, do not drink at all (100% – 56% = 44%) and that (b) the heavier alcohol use

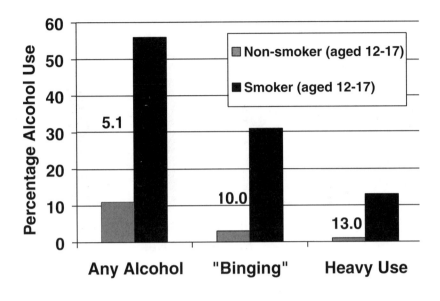

Figure 7.1. Percentage Alcohol Use in the Past Month by 12- to 17-year-olds, by Cigarette Use in the Past Month
SOURCE: National Household Survey, 1998 (Substance Abuse and Mental Health Services Administration, 1999).
NOTE: Added numbers indicate relative risk of alcohol use in smokers compared with nonsmokers. See text for definitions of binging and heavy alcohol use.

categories contain more smokers. (The percentages of alcohol use would be higher in a sample of 17- to 18-year-olds.)

The pattern is somewhat different if the perspective is turned around. If 1 in 10 young smokers is a heavy drinker, what proportion of heavy drinkers are smokers? The answer is also available from the Household Survey: nearly 8 in 10 (see Figure 7.2). In other words, if you drink heavily, you are very likely to be a cigarette smoker. However, many smokers do not drink heavily, although they are more likely to drink heavily than are nonsmokers.

What does the pattern look like if we use more categories of use in both the measure of smoking and the measure of drinking? The relationship between smoking and drinking is seen to be stronger. Figure 7.3 shows data from a survey of schoolchildren in Ontario, Canada (Smart & Adlaf, 1987). Self-reports of getting drunk at least once a month are strongly associated with level of cigarette use. Some 54% of heavy-smoking males (11 to 15 cigarettes per day is heavy smoking

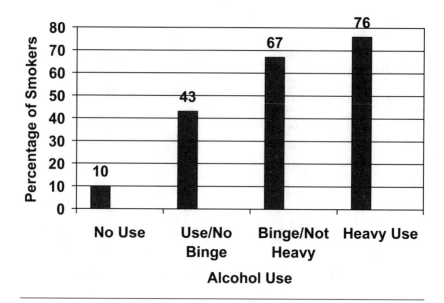

Figure 7.2. Percentage Using Cigarettes in the Past Month as a Function of Alcohol Use in the Past Month for Persons Aged 12-17.
SOURCE: National Household Survey, 1998 (Substance Abuse and Mental Health Services Administration, 1999).

for a teenager still in school) reported getting drunk at least once in the past month. The pattern (not shown) is very similar for females. Figure 7.3 also shows that heavy levels of illicit, nonmedical drug use (a count of 10 substances, including marijuana, barbiturates, stimulants, tranquilizers, heroin, speed, LSD, PCP, other hallucinogens, and cocaine) are more common as smoking levels increase. The basic lesson is that the more that measures of drug-use level are refined, the stronger the association with smoking. The overall pattern in adults is very similar to that found in adolescents.

▇ Substances in Common Use

Scientific surveys of U.S. families consistently find that alcohol and cigarettes are the most frequently used dependence-producing substances in U.S. households, aside from caffeine. In recent years, about half of those aged 12 and older have reported using alcohol within the month prior to being surveyed; about 32% have re-

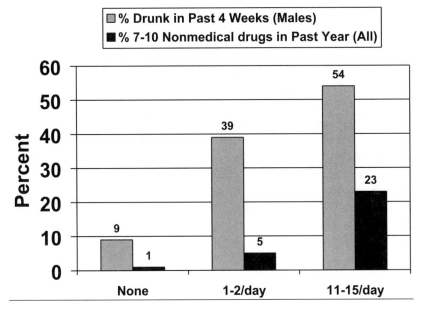

Figure 7.3. Percentage of School Children in Ontario, Canada, Reporting Having Been Drunk in the Past 4 Weeks (for males) or Using 7-10 Nonmedical Drugs in the Past Year, (for males and females combined) by Heaviness of Cigarette Smoking
SOURCE: Secondary analyses from data from Smart and Adlaf (1987).

ported using cigarettes or smokeless tobacco. About 5% have reported using marijuana. Use of all other drugs combined is reported by only about 1% of the respondents. It is important to keep in mind that use of "hard" drugs such as heroin and cocaine is found only within that 1% of respondents and is therefore dramatically less common than alcohol, cigarettes, and caffeine.

Caffeine

Often overlooked in discussions of common drugs of abuse is the everyday component of chocolate, soft drinks, coffee, and tea—caffeine (James, 1997; Strain, Mumford, Silverman, & Griffiths, 1994). Researchers have determined what many daily coffee drinkers know: If they attempt to go a day without their usual dose of caffeine, they typically experience headaches and have difficulty thinking clearly (James, 1997). Some experience nausea and feel physically ill. These symptoms tend to subside within a few days.

Caffeine is readily available virtually worldwide to any person with the spare change it costs to purchase a soft drink or a cup of coffee. Like alcohol, caffeine is frequently used in conjunction with tobacco, and caffeine interacts with tobacco in ways that heighten both the social and the physical experience of using tobacco. About 77% of nonsmokers drink coffee, but the rate of coffee drinking among smokers is 86%, and heavy smokers typically drink more coffee than do light smokers (e.g., Kozlowski, 1976). Chemicals in cigarette smoke (not the nicotine) make caffeine metabolize faster in the body (Joeres et al., 1988). Thus, smokers who quit using tobacco but continue to consume their usual amounts of coffee may find that the caffeine is not passing through their systems as quickly, and so they may experience the effects of a cup of coffee longer than they did when they were smoking. It could be easy for them to "overload" on coffee without realizing it, and they might find themselves feeling even more nervous, anxious, and jittery than they would expect to be as a result of nicotine withdrawal.

Alcohol

Because alcohol and tobacco can be purchased legally by adults in the United States, their widespread use is not surprising. About 4 in every 10 smokers experience some problem with alcohol abuse or dependence during their lifetimes (Nothwehr, Lando, & Bobo, 1995). Looking at the issue from the other side is even more illuminating: About 8 of every 10 alcoholics (e.g., those with alcohol abuse or dependence) smoke. Only about 1 in 10 people in the general population is a heavy smoker; among alcoholics, 7 in 10 are *heavy* smokers (e.g., Kozlowski, Jelinek, & Pope, 1986). Despite the close correspondence between alcohol use and heavy smoking, recent research shows that most alcoholics who quit using alcohol can also quit using tobacco without experiencing a relapse to alcohol use. However, among alcoholics, quitting smoking does not necessarily lead to a reduction in alcohol use (Nothwehr, Lando, & Bobo, 1995).

Both alcohol and tobacco are addictive, and both cause disease and death. Both produce a number of pharmacological effects that lead to their characterization as addictive drugs (see Chapter 6). However, alcohol and tobacco *differ* in some significant ways:

- Tobacco use results in tobacco dependence far more often than drinking alcohol results in alcohol dependence. Only a minority of alcohol users meet the criteria for an alcohol use disorder (e.g., Alcohol Abuse or Alcohol Dependence, as determined by *DSM-IV;* American Psychiatric Association,

1994). Conversely, perhaps 95% of regular users of tobacco can be considered addicted to some degree.

▨ Tobacco use typically does not result in a state of intoxication or inebriation that impairs daily functioning.

▨ Smokers with alcohol problems find that alcohol and cigarettes both produce strong urges for use, but alcohol can produce stronger pleasurable effects than cigarettes (Kozlowski, Wilkinson, et al., 1989).

▨ Smoking and alcohol use are not distributed evenly across the population. Smoking is more prevalent among those of lower education levels and among blue-collar versus white-collar workers. Use of alcohol, on the other hand, tends to cross educational and socioeconomic boundaries.

▨ Abstinence in someone who is dependent on either substance can result in unpleasant or even debilitating withdrawal symptoms. However, in the case of alcohol dependence, these symptoms can include life-threatening seizures.

Use of both substances differs somewhat between the sexes. For this reason, some experts have proposed that men's and women's differing reasons for using both substances and differing experiences in abstinence may warrant different types of interventions (e.g., Nothwehr, Lando, & Bobo, 1995; Perkins, Donny, & Caggiula, 1999; Thomas, 1996). Using both substances together can be particularly dangerous, because the interaction between heavy smoking and excessive drinking escalates the health risk for disease, especially oral cancers.

A research team at the University of Pittsburgh found that, used by itself, nicotine increased sensations such as "head rush," dizziness, and stimulant effects. Alcohol, used by itself, increased intoxication, head rush, dizziness, and jitteriness, but without stimulant effects. Used together, nicotine and alcohol had an additive effect, but nicotine attenuated the sedating and intoxicating effects of alcohol. The effects were somewhat different in men and women, with the combination of the two substances attenuating some of the effects of either substance in men but enhancing the effects of either substance in women (Perkins et al., 1995).

Cigarettes, Caffeine, and Alcohol Together

Samples of drug abusers were studied at the Addiction Research Center in Baltimore and at the Addiction Research Foundation in Toronto (Kozlowski et al., 1993). According to the resulting data, severity of alcoholism was directly related to various measures of tobacco and caffeinated beverage use. These three substances were more strongly related to each other than they were to the use of other drugs of abuse (e.g., heroin, marijuana, or glue). Psychosocial/behavioral factors may account for these findings in that alcohol, tobacco, and cigarettes are all similarly legal and available to adults; however, biological and pharmacological factors may also contribute to the close association of these drugs, as will be discussed below.

Patterns of Sequential Use

Tobacco has been studied for decades as a possible *gateway* substance—a legal and easily obtainable substance whose use is associated with increased risk of using illegal drugs and alcohol. Alcohol itself is sometimes considered a gateway to illicit drug use, and marijuana is often considered a gateway to the use of hard drugs such as heroin and cocaine. The typical developmental pathway involves a sequence of substance use that begins with a relatively easily obtainable substance such as alcohol or tobacco, usually in early adolescence (see Kandel, 1980; Kandel & Yamaguchi, 1985). Some young people then progress to the use of other substances, often including marijuana. Later, some marijuana users use drugs such as opiates or cocaine. The trajectory, however, is not inevitable; not everyone who uses tobacco or alcohol as an adolescent goes on to use marijuana, and not every marijuana user progresses to the use of heroin or cocaine.

The exact course toward substance use that some children and adolescents follow tends to differ somewhat among generations and ethnic groups and between the sexes, varying according to what substances are available and popular in different locales. Nonetheless, the pattern of escalating substance use may be a valid framework for understanding how people go from using no substances to using substances that can destroy their minds and lives. Consider these examples from throughout the world:

> ▶ *Mexican American school children in Texas differed according to grade (e.g., fourth grade, fifth, or sixth) in using cigarettes, beer, wine or liquor, and marijuana. Fourth- and fifth-grade boys and girls differed in their use of these substances, although these differences were less evident for sixth graders (Katims & Zapata, 1993). Smoking in seventh grade by Hispanic students in California (Parra-Medina, Talavera, Elder, & Woodruff, 1995) was strongly linked statistically to the use of alcohol by ninth grade. Not only did smoking in seventh grade statistically "predict" alcohol use, but it*

also was associated with intentions to drink, sexual behavior among girls, and poor grades in school. Smoking among young Hispanics can therefore be seen as a behavior that places them at risk for other illegal and undesirable behaviors (see Jackson, Henriksen, Dickinson, & Levine, 1997).

▸ *Japanese young people, however, are in a somewhat different situation. For them, the inhalation of solvents as a way to get "high" is a sufficiently serious and widespread practice that researchers have examined the roles of cigarette smoking and alcohol use as gateways for solvent inhalation abuse. Findings of Japan's National Institute of Mental Health indicate that cigarette smoking by junior high school students is strongly related to inhaling solvents but that alcohol consumption depends on the presence of adults (Oh, Yamazaki, & Kawata, 1998). This is in contrast to the United States, where alcohol consumption by underage drinkers generally occurs in the presence of peers.*

▸ *A survey of more than 5,000 English adolescents found that substance use increased with age. The prevalence of regular use of tobacco, alcohol, or illicit drugs rose dramatically between age 11 and age 16 (Sutherland & Willner, 1998). Alcohol was the most commonly used substance, with 30% of 11-year-olds reporting that they use alcohol and 83% using it by age 16. Cigarette use appeared to peak among 15-year-olds at 30%. Use of illegal drugs rose from 1% of the sample at age 11 to 32% at age 16. Cigarette smoking was more prevalent in girls than in boys, and boys were more likely to use illicit drugs. Cigarettes or drugs were used in combination with alcohol nearly all of the time. The authors of the study concluded that their findings were consistent with the gateway hypothesis of drug use, although the findings also fit with an alternative approach in which substance use is considered to be a manifestation of a pattern of delinquency.*

Even though the specifics differ from locale to locale and from situation to situation, some general principles apply. The results of dozens of studies indicate that the use of some substances tends to lead to the use of others. In some settings, cigarette use may be a precursor to marijuana and alcohol use. In others, marijuana use may actually lead to cigarette use. These associations also vary by age. Nonetheless, it is clear that the use of tobacco is intertwined with the use of other substances; even if tobacco use does not necessarily lead to other substance use, tobacco is often used in conjunction with other substances. The different trajectories of drug use in different cultural settings is probably not due to biological factors (e.g., differences in genetics) but, rather, to sociocultural factors (e.g., drug availability and beliefs about proper behavior for males and females).

Why Is Smoking Associated With Alcohol and Other Drug Use?

The Addictive Personality?

A common belief is that an addictive personality is responsible for the association between cigarette and other drug use. However, no personality factor has been found that explains the clustering of addictions. Although some personality traits (e.g., extroversion) are somewhat more likely in smokers than nonsmokers, scores overlap considerably. Many nonsmokers are just as extroverted as smokers (U. S. Department of Health Education and Welfare, 1979). Though the addictive personality may seem to account for the patterns of drug use, its value as a scientific explanation never has been demonstrated and may be little more than another way to describe the syndrome of multiple drug use. Some drug researchers view the addictive personality as a completely fruitless concept (Phil & Spiers, 1978).

Connections Between Substances and Vulnerability to Drug Use

Is there a common source of vulnerability to drug abuse? A great deal of contemporary research on drug abuse is directed at exploring and elucidating the bases of individual differences in vulnerability to drug abuse. Some individuals grow up in high-risk settings in which, for example, their friends and immediate family all have serious drug abuse problems, and yet these individuals do not become drug abusers. (Remember, we do categorize cigarette use as a substance abuse problem.) Other individuals come from very low-risk environments and overcome the odds by becoming drug abusers. Environmental factors and genetic factors together influence recruitment to drug use. When speaking of genetic factors, it probably is not true that a single gene influences vulnerability to drug abuse; rather, multiple genetic determinants—several different combinations of genes—are likely to be involved. Groups of genes that affect sensitivity to the negative effects of nicotine (or something else in cigarette smoke) and different groups of genes that influence positive reactions to nicotine all may have distinct genetic influences on smoking behavior (e.g., see Pomerleau, 1995). It is important to also keep in mind that psychosocial factors (e.g., the religion you were born into) can keep you from ever trying a drug, and thus, your genetic-based reactions to drugs never have the opportunity to influence whether you become a drug abuser (Kozlowski, 1991; see also Chapter 4).

A series of studies (Swan, Carmelli, & Cardon, 1996, 1997) exploring the joint use of substances has identified a common genetic substrate. The investigators found two independent sets of multiple genes, or *polygenes,* and hypothesized that the combined use of the substances stems from "the need to respond to an environmental demand with heightened cognitive abilities" (1997, p. 189). For example, the combined use of nicotine and caffeine would enhance alertness, vigilance, and concentration.

Research has also shown that drugs of abuse can change normal physiology in distinct ways. Alterations in stress responses, immune functions, and reproductive biology may be persistent and may influence an individual's reactions to subsequent drug taking (Kreek, 1992). These reactions also may influence the effects of drugs on health (Kreek, 1987).

Laboratory research also provides insight into the relationships between alcohol, caffeine, and tobacco. For example, prolonged exposure to alcohol affects the behavior of mice that are then exposed to nicotine, thus indicating that alcohol use increased the sensitization of the mice to nicotine (Watson & Little, 1999). Similarly, exposing rats to caffeine resulted in the rats' self-administering considerably more nicotine than was self-administered by caffeine-free "control" rats (Shoaib, Swanner, Yasar, & Goldberg, 1999). These findings suggest that caffeine potentiates, or strengthens, the reinforcing properties of nicotine. The mechanisms underlying these effects are not yet well understood. However, Shoaib and colleagues assert that it appears certain that the use of nicotine and caffeine together is "not merely coincidental; rather, smokers who drink coffee may enhance the addictive properties of nicotine in tobacco" (p. 332). The use of caffeine and nicotine also may be linked, not because of direct pharmacological effects but because the withdrawal of one substance can promote the use of the other substance (Kozlowski, 1976).

Perkins and his colleagues (summarized in Perkins, Donny, & Caggiula, 1999) found that differences in the effects of nicotine can also be due to the situations in which nicotine is used. Women may be more sensitive than men to situational factors, such as the sight and taste of cigarette smoke. Perkins and colleagues have also speculated that men and women may smoke for different reasons—men to maintain a steady level of nicotine in their bodies, and women to obtain effects less related to nicotine and more related to the smoking experience itself. The thousands of chemical compounds and the many complex factors associated with smoking can generate additional responses to those produced by nicotine.

It should be noted that the interrelationships among substances of abuse and their patterns of concurrent use can make research difficult. In persons using multiple substances, it can be a challenge to identify the specific effects of the various drugs being used (Kozlowski & Ferrence, 1990). So many alcohol addicts also smoke cigarettes that it is difficult to use statistical procedures to control for the effects of alcohol and act *as if* one had created a valid comparison group of nonsmoking alcoholics.

■ The Concept of Risk

Human activities, often studied in isolation or in a laboratory setting, take on richer dimensions in the varied real-life environments in which people actually smoke a cigarette, have a drink of alcohol, and sip coffee. The aspects of substance use that are teased apart and analyzed by epidemiologists and other scientists are not necessarily perceived by the drug users themselves. Progression from one substance of abuse to another is rarely orderly or consistent, and no statistical prediction of substance use is completely accurate. Our understanding of the influences of one substance on the use of another comes from our ability to analyze behaviors on the broad scale of hundreds and thousands of persons. Using this broad view, we can see that many factors place a person at risk for tobacco, alcohol, and other substance use. However, the presence of those risk factors by no means condemns a person to a life of addiction. Among the many elements that have been identified as risk factors for substance use are these (see also Chapter 5):

- ■ Family history of substance use
- ■ Peer relationships
- ■ Peer acceptance or rejection of substance use
- ■ Depression or other psychiatric condition
- ■ Inadequate parental supervision
- ■ Access to substances such as alcohol
- ■ Awareness of health risks
- ■ Family discord

The concept of *risk* is best applied in a wide sense. A young person is not necessarily at risk for only one substance of abuse or for one type of problematic behavior. Rather, risk is more likely related to complex forces and interactions that can have interwoven consequences and multiply unfortunate outcomes.

Progression in Drug Use

The concept of *progression* is based in part on the observations that the national prevalence of a drug declines to smaller and smaller levels as the drug type is classed as harder; for example, among high school student smokers in the United States, 82% currently used alcohol, 54% used marijuana, and only 7% used cocaine (Everett, Giovino, Warren, Crossett, & Kann, 1998). Although only a fraction of users at any given level also use harder drugs, most individuals at any given level also have regularly used substances in the lower levels. The finding that very few smokers actually go on to use harder drugs is evidence that smoking is not a strong cause of harder drug use; if it were, many more smokers would have moved on to harder drugs.

Although gateway models have some utility, it must be recognized that several aspects of progression are based in part on social attitudes, legal sanctions, and the availability and cost of drugs at any point in time and not necessarily on the pharmacology or toxicology or addictiveness of the drugs (see Chapter 6). The high cost and lack of availability of some drugs, such as heroin, represent barriers that don't come into play with cigarette use. It will be interesting to see how multiple drug use patterns change over the next century as attitudes, availability, policies, and types of drugs and drug delivery systems change.

The opinion of these authors is that cigarette smoking does not meet the causal criteria necessary (see Chapter 3) to be regarded as a *cause* of other drug abuse but is nonetheless more than a simple associated factor. Cigarettes may promote progression to other drug use. This determination has implications for policy and research. On the policy side, it suggests that efforts to reduce illicit drug abuse that aim to reduce the demand for drugs by offering treatment alternatives, as well as alternative activities (e.g., youth centers, safe playgrounds, and recreational centers, and job training), should also include prevention of cigarette smoking. Prevention programs are important not because smoking prevention will solve the drug abuse problem but because smoking cigarettes is one of the many factors that appear to contribute to the overall prevalence of heavy drinking and illicit drug abuse.

Summary

Compared with nonsmokers, smokers are more likely to use psychoactive substances. And heavy smokers are more likely to use psychoactive substances than are light smokers. Both biological and behavioral factors determine the interrelationships of drugs of abuse. A host of factors contributes to vulnerability to substance use—some genetic, some cultural, some psychosocial. Smoking is best viewed more as a *risk factor* than a *causative step* relative to the use of other substances.

Further Reading

Kandel, D. B., & Yamaguchi, K. (1985). Developmental patterns of the use of legal, illegal, and medically prescribed psychotropic drugs from adolescence to young adulthood. In C. L. Jones & R. J. Battjes (Eds.), *Etiology of drug abuse: Implications for prevention* (DHHS Publication No. ADM 85-1335, pp. 193-235). Washington, DC: Government Printing Office.

This is a classic study on progression in drug use.

Kozlowski, L. T., Henningfield, J. E., Keenan, R. M., Lei, H., Leigh, G., Jelinek, L., Pope, M. A., & Haertzen, C. A. (1993). Patterns of alcohol, cigarette, and caffeine and other drug use in two drug abusing populations. *Journal of Substance Abuse Treatment, 10,* 171-179.

This study reviews drug use patterns among patients and research participants at the U.S. National Institute of Drug Abuse Addiction Research Center and the Addiction Research Foundation of Ontario, Canada.

Swan, G. E., Carmelli, D., & Cardon, L. R. (1996). The consumption of tobacco, alcohol, and coffee in Caucasian male twins: A multivariate genetic analysis. *Journal of Substance Abuse, 8,* 19-31.

An excellent example of research on genetic-based patterns in drug use.

8

"Low-Tar," "Light" Cigarettes

Lessons From a Dangerous Boondoggle

The cigarette that takes the FEAR out of smoking.

—Advertising slogan, Philip Morris Cigarettes, 1954

Wherever the disease risks of smoking are well-known, filtered cigarettes or lower-tar and lower-nicotine cigarettes are promoted as less hazardous or safer. It seems sensible that, if tar is bad for a smoker, then a cigarette that produces less tar would be less harmful both to the individual smoker and society. Low-tar cigarettes (< 15 mg standard tar) are now the best-selling cigarettes in the United States. Nonetheless, the low-tar cigarette is a boondoggle—a scam—that gives smokers a false sense of security and keeps many health-conscious smokers from trying to quit smoking.

Cigarettes are called "low-tar" and "light" largely because of a deeply flawed testing and labeling system. This standard test does not measure the tar and nicotine actually *contained* in a cigarette but merely shows how much tar and nicotine result when a cigarette is smoked in one fixed way—a way that cannot represent the many varieties of human smoking behaviors. The disease risks of smoking were not substantially reduced by the introduction of low-yield cigarettes; the cigarette is a sophisticated drug delivery system carefully designed to be maximally addictive. Marketing strategies help keep smokers smoking despite all the publicity about smoking and disease.

■ A Less Hazardous Alternative?

Lung cancer was rare during the first decades of the 20th century in the United States. It took decades of people inhaling cigarette smoke to create lung cancer as a public health problem. At that time, cigar and pipe smokers were concerned that their tobacco use would lead to oral or throat cancer (Patterson, 1989). A popular model of what caused cancer was the *irritation* model. According to this model, excessive use of tobacco irritated the delicate tissues of the throat and mouth and thus ultimately caused cancer. Smoke-based irritation of the throat and mouth from strong pipe and cigar tobaccos was believed to cause oral and throat cancers. Compared with cigars and pipes, "milder," "less irritating" cigarettes were viewed as a much safer way to use tobacco. Scientists now know that this model of vulnerability was inaccurate.

The slogans of the early national advertising campaigns for cigarettes were designed to allay smokers' fears that cigarettes would (a) irritate the mouth or throat, (b) cause ill health, (c) be impure (e.g., be contaminated with filthy or dangerous substances), and (d) be used immoderately or excessively. Camel cigarettes were once promoted by indicating, "You never tasted such mellow-mildness . . . And, you can smoke Camels as liberally as meets your wishes, for they never tire your taste." Later, an ad said, "More Doctors Smoke Camels Than Any Other Cigarette." Of Lucky Strike it was said, "It's toasted," and "No Throat Irritation—No cough." Another ad claimed that "20,679 physicians have confirmed the fact that Lucky Strike is less irritating in the throat than other cigarettes." Some ads for Old Gold cigarettes read, "OLD GOLD cigarettes, better . . . smoother . . . not a cough in a carload."

A "good" cigarette was "pleasant" in that it produced positive drug effects on the central nervous system and positive stimulation of taste and smell. A good cigarette also was viewed as *not dangerous*. For cigarettes, perceived safety has been a function of the cleanness or purity of the smoke and the excessiveness of its use. Terms such as *light, mellow,* and *smooth* were especially potent descriptive claims in that they addressed smokers' concerns about purity and excessiveness while at the same time implying safety without having to claim it explicitly (Kozlowski, 2000).

▧ Tar Derby

Product modification was a response of the cigarette industry to the health consequences of smoking. *Tar Derby* refers to the race in the 1950s by cigarette manufacturers in the United States to create and market lower- and lower-tar cigarettes (e.g., see Brecher, 1967). If one of your favorite foods was found to be dangerous, wouldn't you be trying to find a version of the food that had removed or at least decreased the dangerous or undesirable ingredients? Does the strategy sound familiar: *light* ice cream, *diet* colas, *low-fat* foods?

The formerly secret documents of the cigarette industry are revealing in this regard. Cohen (1992) reviewed company marketing analyses as part of a court case in Canada. He reported that lower-tar cigarettes were being promoted to help keep health-concerned smokers smoking. In 1976, Ernest Pepples, vice president and general counsel for Brown & Williamson Tobacco Company, wrote a memo, titled, "Industry Response to Cigarette/Health Controversy" (Glantz, Slade, Bero, Hanauer, & Barnes, 1996). He noted that "the 'tar derby' in the United States resulted from industry efforts to cater to the public's concern"(p. 254).

As the public became more and more aware of the health risks of smoking, smokers turned to lower-tar and filtered cigarettes to reduce risks to their health. In 1967 when standardized testing for tar and nicotine began in the United States, only 2% of all cigarettes sold were considered low tar (that is, 15 mg standard tar or less); by 1996, two thirds (67%) of cigarettes sold were considered low tar (Federal Trade Commission [FTC], 1997).

Smokers may have the inaccurate impression that the governmental attention to cigarette smoke and its dangers has led to cigarettes' becoming less dangerous. Figure 8.1 shows the sales-weighted standard tar yields from 1968 through 1997. Although standard tar dropped a substantial 39% (8.4 mg) from 1968 to 1981, thereafter, standard yields dropped little (9%, 1.2 mg). The dashed line in Figure 8.1 indicates what standard tar yields would have been had the decreasing pattern of yields from 1968 to 1981 continued. The popularity of very low tar cigarettes

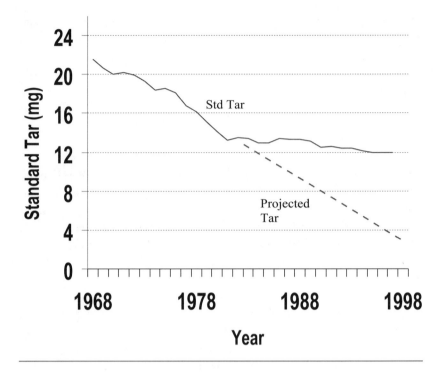

Figure 8.1. Sales-Weighted Standard Tar Yield
SOURCE: Reports to Congress of the Federal Trade Commission, 1968-1998.
NOTE: Projected values (estimated by authors) are shown by dashed line, indicating the drop that would have been expected based on the drop that was seen until the early 1980s.

appears limited. Despite industry efforts to advertise and promote the lowest-tar cigarettes (1-3 mg), sales remained low (Kozlowski, 1989), perhaps because smoking these cigarettes in a satisfying way can be hard work.

▪ Why Smoke Lower-Tar Cigarettes?

Smokers cite many reasons for choosing light (> 6-15 mg standard tar) or ultra-light (< 6 mg standard tar) cigarettes; the most problematic reasons relate to the belief that these cigarettes will reduce the dangers of smoking. Figure 8.2 shows the results of a recent national survey of daily smokers of light and ultra-light cigarettes. Respondents were asked to endorse reasons for smoking these cigarettes. Those who smoked ultra-lights endorsed a greater percentage of health-related

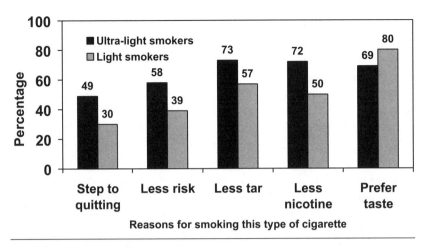

Figure 8.2. Perceived Reasons for Smoking Light and Ultra Light Cigarettes From a National Sample of Smokers in the United States
SOURCE: Data from Kozlowski, Goldberg, et al. (1998).

reasons than did those who smoked lights. Some 58% of ultra-lights smokers and 39% of lights smokers reported smoking brands "to reduce the risks of smoking without having to give up smoking" (Kozlowski, Goldberg, et al., 1998). Clearly, a high percentage of smokers of these lower-tar cigarettes are expecting less tar and less nicotine.

Why don't 100% of smokers say they smoke lower-tar cigarettes to reduce the risks of smoking? Health concerns are not the only reason for smoking lower-tar cigarettes. Brand popularity also influences brand selection. Because lights have become the best-selling cigarettes, this increases the likelihood that an individual is smoking lights because others smoke lights, not because of hopes about reducing exposure to toxins.

In summary, it is clear that a substantial percentage of consumers think that light and ultra-light cigarettes reduce risks to human smokers (Giovino et al., 1996; Kozlowski et al., 1999; Kozlowski, Goldberg, et al., 1998; Kozlowski, Rickert, Pope, Robinson, & Frecker, 1982; Rickert, Robinson, & Lawless, 1989).

Standard Tar Yield Results: Misleading

To understand why lower-tar cigarettes have, at best, a limited impact on health risk, it is helpful to understand the standard smoking-machine test for tar and nicotine yields. Although exact procedures for testing cigarettes vary somewhat from country to country (and many developing countries do not do cigarette testing), the procedures for U.S. Federal Trade Commission testing are representative (Peeler, 1996).

Figure 8.3 depicts the standard test, which provides the criteria for producing what can be labeled as a lower-tar and lower-nicotine cigarette. The only official definition of the lower-yield cigarette is that it gives lower tar and nicotine yields in this smoking-machine test. The roots of this smoking-machine test have little to do with human smoking behavior. In the 1930s, a major cigarette manufacturer developed this testing procedure to compare one tobacco crop with another (Bradford, Harlan, & Hanmer, 1936). Such crop testing did not need to simulate or model human smoking behavior precisely. The standard test involves a "smoking machine" taking a 35-ml, 2-second duration puff once each minute. A 35-ml puff is less than that drawn in by human smokers, who typically take in 40 to 50 ml of smoke. More important than the average amount, however, is the range of individual puff sizes. Some smokers take small puffs (e.g., 15 ml) and some take much larger puffs (e.g., 120 ml). From start to stop of each puff, a machine takes 2 seconds. A human smoker taking a larger puff in 2 seconds increases the velocity of the puff. A 60-ml puff in 2 seconds yields 30 ml of smoke per second, as opposed to 17.5 ml of smoke per second in a standard machine puff. Higher puff velocities decrease filter efficiency. The *efficiency* of the cigarette filter refers to the percentage of presented smoke caught by the filter: The higher the percentage of smoke caught by the filter, the higher the filter's efficiency.

The official tests involve 1 puff per minute. Human smokers often puff more frequently, and the puffing rate changes as the needs of the smoker change. Human smokers easily can puff once each 20 seconds. In these and other aspects, human smoking behavior is highly variable (U. S. Department of Health and Human Services [USDHHS], 1988). The cigarette industry has designed cigarettes to give lower tar numbers on the standard test and higher tar numbers when smoked by smokers (Kozlowski & O'Connor, 2000).

■ Making a Low-Yield Cigarette

A lower-yield cigarette can cause fewer puffs to be taken per cigarette and can cause less smoke to be delivered by each puff (i.e., reduce the concentration of smoke per puff) when smoked on a smoking machine—while allowing human smokers to obtain more puffs and higher smoke concentrations (Kozlowski,

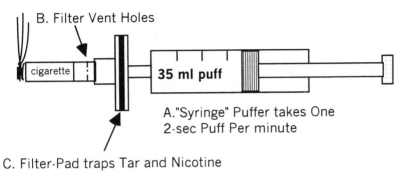

Figure 8.3. A Schematic Drawing of a Basic Smoking Machine

NOTE: The syringe puffer (A) draws smoke from the cigarette—one 2-sec, 35-ml puff every minute until a fixed butt length is left. A major design feature of most modern cigarettes is vents or air-dilution holes on the cigarette filter (B). Air is drawn through the vents to reduce the smoke getting through the cigarette. A filter-pad (C) traps smoke for analysis. "Tar" is basically measured as the change in weight of the filter as a result of smoking cigarettes.

1981). To look into this further, we will first deal with how cigarettes produce lower tar and nicotine yields on smoking machines. This is accomplished in different ways.

Reducing the Number of Puffs per Cigarette

A smoking machine takes one puff per minute on all cigarettes it tests, which results in different cigarettes having different numbers of total puffs drawn by smoking machines (Kozlowski, 1981). One test of popular cigarettes showed that the smoking machines took only 6.9 puffs on some ultra-low-tar brands but took as many a 14 puffs on higher-tar brands (Jenkins, Quincey, & Guerin, 1979). Some historical reductions in advertised tar and nicotine yields were the result of product modifications designed to make the smoking machines take fewer puffs per cigarette (Kozlowski, Rickert, Robinson, & Grunberg, 1980). The cigarette can be manufactured so that a smoking machine will test it with fewer puffs; this is done by making the cigarette shorter, making the cigarette burn faster between puffs. Cigarette makers also can affect smoking machine measurements by manipulating the chemical content or porosity of the cigarette paper or by making the tobacco column less dense by decreasing the weight per volume of tobacco. Tobacco can be puffed up to increase volume in essentially the same way that breakfast cereal can be puffed up.

An apt comparison can be made between eating ice cream and smoking a cigarette. If eating an ice cream cone on a hot day, one can eat faster to finish eating the ice cream before it melts. Similarly, a nicotine-hungry smoker can compensate for a cigarette that burns more quickly by taking puffs more quickly.

Reducing the Concentration of Smoke in Each Puff

Diluting the smoke with air reduces the concentration of smoke in each puff. Increasing the porosity of the cigarette paper increases air dilution, as does adding ventilation holes to a filter. Filter ventilation has been an increasingly important design feature in cigarettes. Filter ventilation generally increases as tar yields decrease. At present, most U.S. cigarettes have ventilated filters. "Full-flavor" cigarettes (e.g., Marlboro®) are slightly ventilated; most, if not all, light and ultralight cigarettes have ventilated filters. On 1-mg tar cigarettes (the lowest-yield cigarettes), ventilation levels can produce 70% to 90% air dilution, which means that each puff a smoking machine takes is diluted 70% to 90% with air. Although various manufacturing changes have contributed to the development of lower-tar and lower-nicotine cigarettes, filter ventilation has been the major change behind the modern "low-yield" cigarettes (Kozlowski, Mehta, Sweeney, Richter, & Giovino, 1997; Kozlowski, Mehta, et al., 1998).

■ How Smokers Compensate

The actual tar and nicotine yield of a cigarette—as it is consumed by a smoker—depends mainly on smoking behaviors such as puff duration, puff volume, and puff frequency. Therefore, reductions in machine-smoked standard tar and nicotine yields are often not reflected in changes in tar and nicotine exposures in smokers (Gerstein & Levison, 1982; Participants of the Fourth Scarborough Conference on Preventive Medicine, 1985; Scherer, 1999). Smokers easily compensate for reduced yields by changing the way they smoke each cigarette by doing the following:

■ Taking bigger puffs
■ Taking more puffs
■ Smoking more cigarettes per day
■ Blocking filter vent holes on heavily ventilated (> 70%), very low tar cigarettes (about 1 mg tar)

Blocking filter ventilation holes increases smoke exposure by reducing the filter air dilution. For moderately ventilated cigarettes (about 60% dilution or less), increasing puff volumes can make blocking ventilation holes with the lips or the finger, unnecessary (Kozlowski, O'Connor, & Sweeney, in press). Blocking appears to be an important mode of compensation for smokers of the lowest-yield cigarettes (1 mg tar, about 80% diluted) but not for higher-yield cigarettes (Sweeney, Kozlowski, & Parsa, 1999). Both blocking the ventilation holes and taking bigger puffs may be outside the smoker's awareness.

Recently released tobacco industry documents support the assertion that nearly invisible vents may have been part of a research-and-development strategy for some manufacturers. In a British American Tobacco document ("R & D Views on Potential Marketing Opportunities," Pangritz, 1984), Point 1, titled, "Elastic/Compensatible Products," in a section labeled "high priority," notes: "Irrespective of the ethics involved, we should develop alternative designs (that do not invite obvious criticism) which allow the smoker to obtain significant enhanced deliveries should he so wish." Most smokers are unaware of blocking ventilation holes and are unaware of the consequences of blocking for tar and nicotine yields (Kozlowski, Rickert, et al., 1982; Kozlowski, Goldberg, et al., 1997; Kozlowski, White, et al., 1998).

One of the best studies on smoker compensation for lower-nicotine cigarettes was conducted by tobacco industry scientists (Byrd, Davis, Caldwell, Robinson, & deBethizy, 1997) who found no differences in nicotine exposures among 1 mg tar (the lowest tar), ultra-light cigarettes, or light cigarettes. Thus, for cigarettes with standard tar yields ranging from 1 to 11 mg tar, nicotine exposure does not differ. These scientists did find that "full-flavor" cigarettes deliver somewhat higher levels of nicotine than do the other categories of cigarettes; but we think there is little reason to believe that this small difference has any effect on health.

As should be evident by now, cigarettes are highly engineered devices that enable cigarette smokers to have considerable flexibility in getting the dose of nicotine that their bodies crave—regardless of the nicotine delivery rating of the Federal Trade Commission and regardless of whether the cigarette brand is advertised as light or low tar. We have just discussed some of the ways that smokers can compensate for the design alterations of brands advertised as reduced delivery. Such a discussion might appear to lay the blame for compensation fully at the feet of the nicotine-addicted smoker. But a closer examination of the design features and tobacco industry documents shows that cigarette design does more than just enable a person smoking a so-called light brand to obtain more nicotine and tar than advertised: Several aspects of the design features make it virtually inevitable. As discussed earlier, the use and placement of invisible ventilation holes is one such feature, but there are many more.

In its investigation of cigarette-manufacturing practices, the U.S. Food and Drug Administration (FDA, 1996) showed that cigarette manufacturers go to extraordinary lengths to support advertising that makes claims such as "you don't have to sacrifice taste in a light cigarette," in marketing cigarettes that almost inevitably provide more taste—and more tar and more nicotine than implied by the advertised level. For example, the use of ammonia additives in cigarettes results in more absorbable nicotine being delivered to the smoker than is implied by the FTC ratings (Bates, Connolly, & Jarvis, 1999). The use of burn accelerants in the tobacco paper means that a machine might only take 7 or 8 puffs of smoke because so much of the tobacco spontaneously burns during the 1-minute intervals between the machine's programmed puffs. Human cigarette smokers take more frequent puffs, and thus less of the tobacco is spontaneously burned, meaning that the human might take several extra puffs. And these extra puffs are highly concentrated in tar and nicotine. As shown in documents from the tobacco industry itself, such cigarette design features were intended to provide smokers with higher levels of tar and nicotine than implied by the advertising (Hurt & Robertson, 1998; Slade & Henningfield, 1998).

Do Low-Tar Cigarettes Reduce Risks to Health?

The sales-weighted standard tar yields of cigarettes dropped from an estimated 38 mg tar in the mid-1960s to 12 mg tar in the 1990s (Hoffman & Hoffman, 1997). It would seem that such a large reduction in cigarette tar should reduce premature death from cigarette smoking. Early evidence indicated that lower-tar cigarettes decreased disease. An American Cancer Society study of 1 million persons compared people who smoked high-tar cigarettes with those who smoked low-tar cigarettes. One of the main findings was that for every 100 deaths of smokers of a high-tar cigarette, 81 deaths resulted among smokers of lower-tar cigarettes (Hammond, Garfinkel, Seidman, & Lew, 1976). Although some people attributed the differences in mortality to the differences in standard tar yields, there are many possible reasons for the difference (Royal College of Physicians, 2000; USDHHS, 1989). Lower-tar smokers are generally more health conscious and are better educated (Royal College of Physicians, 2000). Moreover, even if there was some appearance of reduced risks from lower-tar cigarettes, this does not justify reduced efforts to encourage smoking cessation, because the benefits of stopping smoking are much greater than the proposed benefits of lower-tar cigarettes. Also, lower-tar cigarettes have not been demonstrated to lower the risk of smoking-related cardiovascular disease (USDHHS, 1989).

Recently, Burns, Shanks, Major, and Thun (in press) have reanalyzed the original American Cancer Society data and concluded that the original analyses were marred by conceptual errors. Because lower-tar smokers tended to smoke more cigarettes per day, statistical adjustments made lower-tar cigarettes seem less dangerous. Using improved analytic techniques, Burns and Shanks found no evidence of reduced mortality associated with lower-tar cigarettes. Thun, Day-Lally, Calle, Flanders, and Heath (1995) have found that modern lower-tar cigarettes have changed the type of lung cancer that smokers are contracting. An increase in adenocarcenoma has been attributed to the deeper inhalation promoted by the milder-tasting smoke from ventilated filter cigarettes.

Even a small reduction in disease risk from lower-tar cigarettes does not offset the effects of these cigarettes on the likelihood of quitting (Warner & Slade, 1992). About 30% of smokers say they would try to quit smoking if they learned that one light cigarette gave them as much tar as one regular cigarette (Kozlowski, Goldberg, et al., 1998). As intended, light cigarettes appear to be reducing motivation for smokers to quit smoking. The fact remains that the best way for a smoker to reduce the disease risks of smoking is to stop smoking.

Summary

The lower-tar cigarette has been the main response of the cigarette industry to concerns about smoking and health. Lower-tar cigarettes have become the best-selling cigarettes. Lower-tar cigarettes are defined by a misleading standard based on a problematic smoking-machine test. Because of compensatory smoking, smokers continue to receive the same amount of tar and nicotine from cigarettes. However, now smokers consume more cigarettes, take bigger or more frequent puffs, and, on the lowest-tar cigarettes, block filter ventilation holes with their lips or fingers. Recent, improved analyses of data from one of the largest studies on the mortality risks of low-yield cigarettes find no evidence of risk reduction from smoking lower-tar cigarettes.

Further Reading

Burns, D., Shanks, T., Major, J., & Thun, M. (in press). Evidence on disease risks in public health consequences of low yield cigarettes. In *Smoking and Tobacco Control Monograph, 13*. Washington, DC: National Cancer Institute.

A reanalysis of a historic data set.

Glantz, S. A., Slade, J., Bero, L. A., Hanauer, P., & Barnes, D. E. (1996). *The cigarette papers.* Berkeley: University of California Press.

A fascinating analysis of formerly secret cigarette industry documents.

Kozlowski, L. T., O'Connor, R., & Sweeney, C. T. (in press). Cigarette design. *Smoking and Tobacco Control Monograph, 13.* Washington, DC: National Cancer Institute.

This review essay describes the design of lower-tar cigarettes and makes use of industry documents.

Kozlowski, L. T., Heatherton, T. F., Frecker, R. C., & Nolte, H. E. (1989). Self-selected blocking of vents on low-yield cigarettes. *Pharmacology, Biochemistry and Behavior, 33,* 815-819.

This article emphasizes the issue of individual differences in compensatory smokers and reminds us that smokers are not randomly assigned to the brands they use. A few of those smokers who prefer very low-tar cigarettes do so because they desire only a little nicotine.

9

Helping Smokers Quit

We cannot simply stand by and count the dead.

—World Health Organization to House of
Commons, United Kingdom, 2000

Is Quitting Worth It?

A 1997 report confirmed what many people already dreaded: Longtime smokers may experience a biological change that permanently increases their risk for lung cancer. Even those who quit smoking cigarettes and do not smoke for many years are still at risk (American Council on Science and Health [ACSH], 1997). Findings indicate that smoking can cause a series of genetic changes in the lungs that accumulate over time and ultimately lead to lung cancer (Wiencke et al., 1999).

If disease may be inevitable anyway, why quit?

And if a smoker is still young, why quit now? Why not go ahead and enjoy tobacco for a few more years, then quit later, when the health risk is greater?

Several reasons. First, even smokers who have used tobacco for only a short time experience ill effects. Adolescent smokers, for instance, typically already have some airway obstruction and slowed lung growth. Damage to DNA and body organs (particularly the lungs) begins with the first few cigarettes and accumulates across the smoking life span (Wiencke et al., 1999).

It is never too early, and never too late, to quit using tobacco. Stopping smoking at any age reduces the risk of disease attributed to smoking, and the benefits are greater the earlier one stops. For example, quitting before age 50 reduces one's risk of contracting smoking-related diseases by up to 50% (U. S. Department of Health and Human Services [USDHHS], 1990), and the earlier one stops, the lower one's risk for future development of disease. The changes brought about by quitting can begin immediately. Within just one day of quitting smoking, a former smoker's levels of carbon monoxide can be as low as those of a person who has never smoked. As health increases, so does the capacity of the immune system to ward off disease. The body's capacity to heal also increases. Precancerous mouth lesions often disappear when tobacco use ends. The risk of myocardial infarction declines within months after a smoker quits, eventually approaching risk levels of nonsmokers (USDHHS, 1990).

Consider this scenario:

> *A college athlete goes to the dentist for a checkup and a cleaning. After the dental hygienist cleans the young man's teeth, she asks him if he uses tobacco. "Sometimes," he replies. "Not very often." She makes a note on his dental chart—circling the word* current *next to the question, Tobacco use? She also makes a note that the dentist reads carefully when she comes in the room to check the young man's teeth.*
>
> *"I think it's important for you to quit using tobacco," the dentist says, "and we can help you."*
>
> *The athlete argues, almost. "Well, I don't use that much, really. I smoke cigarettes on weekends and use some snuff."*
>
> *"Then the fact that you don't use that much might make it a little easier for you to quit," she counters. "Are you willing to quit using tobacco at this time?"*
>
> *He thinks for several long seconds. A tin of snuff is in his backpack—he didn't use any that morning because he knew he was coming in, and he's ready to use a dip as soon as he gets away from the dentist's office. This weekend, he's planning to get together with friends, who typically all drink beer and smoke cigarettes.*

"Right now might not be a good time," he says. "There's a lot going on." A big game Friday, a party this weekend, a couple of tests next week, a term paper next week—not a good time to think about quitting.

The dentist swings her chair around to look straight at him.

"As your dentist, and as someone who's responsible for advising you about your health, I need to tell you that quitting tobacco is the most important thing you can do to protect your current and future health. You need to know that you have a condition called leukoplakia, which can lead to oral cancer. You also need to know that oral cancer is very deadly and moves very quickly once it starts. It kills half the people who get it.

"You don't have it yet, but you could get it. Believe me, this is more important than whatever it is that makes this a bad time for you to quit using tobacco." She continues, "Can you tell me what makes this a bad time to quit? Maybe we can help you deal with some of those things."

"You'll think they're dumb reasons," he says. "Anyway, all I use is a little snuff and a few cigarettes. I didn't know anything was really wrong with that."

"It could be, if you don't quit," she replies. "We can talk some more about it. Are you ready to let us help you quit?"

He isn't ready, he knows that. But then again, who is ready?

"I don't know," he says. "Let me think about it."

This scenario is becoming increasingly common, and is now an accepted—and, in many instances, expected—part of health care practice throughout the United States. Every visit with a care practitioner, whether the practitioner is a dentist, physician, pharmacist, nurse, social worker, psychologist, or other health care professional, can provide an opportunity to assess tobacco use, to advise tobacco users to quit, and to provide advice and encouragement (Fiore et al., 2000; Raw, McNeill, & West, 1998; Tomasello, 1997; Wetter et al., 1998). New methods and medications make quitting a potentially more successful experience than ever and increase the likelihood that those who quit will be able to stay abstinent (Hughes, in press). As is evident from the example, however, motivation to quit is not automatic, even for those confronted with the health consequences of using tobacco.

An important realization for those considering quitting is that total abstinence is essential (ACSH, 1997; *Smoking Kills,* 1998; USDHHS, 1988). Cutting

back by switching brands or reducing the amount of smoking might actually introduce new health risks (see Chapter 7). Smokers can even dramatically reduce the
number of cigarettes they smoke each day (e.g., from 40 cigarettes to just 10) and
still compensate fully for this by smoking each cigarette much more intensely
(Benowitz, Jacob, Kozlowski, & Yu, 1986). No amount of tobacco use is safe.
Quitting means stopping, completely, for good. The initial attempt to quit, however difficult it may be, is not necessarily the biggest hurdle tobacco users face; for
many, the greatest challenge is avoiding a relapse.

■ Experiencing Withdrawal

Why is quitting so difficult? A major reason many tobacco users find the quitting
process noxious is the *withdrawal symptoms* most smokers experience once they
no longer obtain their usual daily dose of nicotine (Hughes & Hatsukami, 1986).
As the level of nicotine in their blood drops, they experience some constellation
of the following symptoms: anxiety, irritability, difficulty concentrating, restlessness, impatience, hunger, tremors, racing heart, sweating, dizziness, nicotine
craving, sleep disturbance, headache, digestive disturbance, and depression. It is
also common for the ex-smoker to experience increased feelings of aggression
and craving for sweets and to gain a few pounds in the days and weeks immediately following smoking cessation, although this can be moderated with the use of
nicotine-replacement medicine such as nicotine gum (e.g., Dale et al., 1998).

Exactly which of these symptoms a former tobacco user will experience, and
in what order, varies considerably. Also, the symptoms tend to change over time,
with some symptoms emerging soon after the beginning of abstinence, others
coming and going for perhaps 2 weeks, and others lingering for a month or longer.
As many ex-smokers know, urges to smoke and cravings for cigarettes can occur
months and years after one quits smoking (Hughes & Hatsukami, 1986).

The reason for using nicotine replacement (e.g., gum, patch, or inhaler) is to
help curb the worst of these withdrawal symptoms during the high-risk period immediately after becoming abstinent. For many smokers, particularly those who
are dependent on large amounts of nicotine, using nicotine replacement does not
eliminate the withdrawal symptoms entirely, but it reduces them to a manageable
level. For this reason, using nicotine replacement can provide a way for a smoker
to deal with the behaviors associated with smoking—such as smoking while
drinking alcohol with friends—while limiting withdrawal symptoms. Once the

ex-smoker has sufficiently restructured his or her life around the absence of to-bacco, then he or she can taper off the nicotine replacement. At least, that is the ideal scenario for using nicotine replacement products to help deal with tobacco addiction.

Using nicotine replacement is not the same experience as smoking (see Chapter 4). No form of nicotine replacement delivers nicotine as quickly as does smoking; even so, nicotine in gum form delivers nicotine quickly enough that a newly abstinent smoker will begin to experience a fading of withdrawal symp-toms within a few moments. Nicotine is delivered more slowly from the nicotine patch.

Obtaining nicotine from smoked tobacco is a highly reinforced behavior, be-cause the nicotine reaches the brain within a matter of seconds, triggering a com-bination of emotional, cognitive, and physical responses. This positive-reinforce-ment quality of smoked tobacco (using the term *reinforcement* as it is used in the behavioral sciences) is a powerful means of keeping people smoking, because quitting tobacco use involves abandoning this highly reinforced behavior (see Chapters 4 and 5). Thus, the smoker who is quitting faces not only the likelihood of unpleasant withdrawal symptoms but also the loss of effects that the smoker ex-periences as beneficial—for example, the cognitive, emotional, and physical en-hancement provided by nicotine (see review in Benowitz, 1998a).

It is not surprising that a person quitting smoking is far more likely to fail at the attempt than to succeed (e.g., Garvey, Bliss, Hitchcock, Heinhold, & Rosner, 1992; Giovino, Shelton, & Schooley, 1993). Tobacco users come to rely on nico-tine to maintain their normal state of functioning. They rely on it to help them stay alert, relax, feel at ease in social situations, think more clearly, and stay a few pounds slimmer than they would be otherwise. They are not only addicted to nico-tine; they have come to rely on it. In addition, over time, a smoker's idiosyncratic actions of tapping, lighting, and smoking a cigarette become part of a habitual be-havioral repertoire that is difficult to alter. In short, tobacco becomes woven into the smoker's day-to-day living. Quitting tobacco can feel like ripping out an inte-gral part of their lives.

The Threat of Relapse

Because using tobacco can be such an integral part of daily life, creating a tobacco-free life is challenging for someone who has been tobacco dependent. Many situations and events can trigger a relapse. These typically include being in social situations in which others are using tobacco; experiencing sudden, unexpected stress or anxiety; feeling depression or other negative emotions; or perceiving a need for tobacco as a way to cope. Sometimes a relapse is triggered by something that reminds the former user of life with tobacco, such as smelling someone else's tobacco smoke, having a cup of coffee with friends, or staying up late at night to study for an exam. All of these conditions can lead to a single *lapse* episode, which then easily becomes a full-blown *relapse.*

Helping a tobacco-dependent person prepare to change behavior and avoid relapse is a primary goal of treatment (e.g., Miller & Rollnick, 1991). For example, a smoker can help avoid the risk of returning to smoking in social situations by limiting alcohol use while quitting smoking, because drinking alcohol is associated with relapse. Also, living with a continuing smoker lessens the chance that an attempt to quit will be successful. It may be helpful for smokers who share living quarters to quit together or at least make arrangements so that the quitting smoker is not tempted toward relapse by another's smoking. Those planning to quit smoking can find it helpful to discuss these and other situations that present a significant risk for relapse. Through behavioral treatment and groups, quitting smokers can rehearse coping strategies and actions that will help prevent relapse.

■ How to Quit

Many hundreds of research studies from all over the world have examined the process of quitting tobacco, sometimes with a goal of finding a single key, answer, or solution. Searching for the most effective way to quit using tobacco is somewhat akin to searching for the Holy Grail: some researchers believe it's there, but they don't know where to find it. At present, the best approach appears to involve including a variety of components that are individually effective, with the net effect being stronger than the sum of the parts. For example, a stop-smoking program might involve the use of nicotine replacement, a prescription for the medication bupropion, behavioral treatment, group discussions, and individual counseling (Hughes, Goldstein, Hurt, & Shiffman, 1999). However, for some persons, such as adolescents, programs that offer stop-smoking assistance might be hard to find, despite high rates of smoking among adolescents (Tyas & Pederson, 1998). Also, for users of smokeless tobacco, cigars, or other forms of tobacco, few programs are available to help the dependent user quit.

Women Smokers

Some of the many differences between men and women may make it more difficult for women to quit smoking than for men to quit (Perkins, Donny, & Caggiula, 1999). Women tend to experience the physical effects of nicotine differently than men do, and women are more affected than men by external factors such as the smell of smoke and the social setting. Women also tend to worry more about gaining weight when they quit smoking, and women often report starting and maintaining smoking as a way of controlling weight. Nonetheless, women smokers can help keep their children away from secondhand smoke if they themselves will quit. Also, women should not smoke during pregnancy, because smoking while pregnant can result in cognitive deficits and behavioral problems in their offspring, in addition to low birth weight and numerous other health problems (Windsor, Boyd, & Orleans, 1998). In short, it is important that women and girls of all ages avoid and quit tobacco use.

Smokeless Tobacco

The upsurge in the use of smokeless tobacco in the 1980s and 1990s, mostly by young men, eventually led many smokeless users into smoking, but it also resulted in millions of persons remaining dependent on smokeless tobacco (Hatsukami & Severson, 1999; USDHHS, 1986). Quitting smokeless tobacco typically results in some withdrawal symptoms, although these differ slightly from those experienced by smokers who quit using cigarettes. Few programs have addressed the needs of smokeless tobacco users for help in quitting. Some self-help programs have met with success, but such aids as nicotine gum have not been as useful with smokeless users as with smokers. This may be related to findings that smokeless users experience different effects from tobacco than smokers experience.

Avoiding Weight Gain

Using tobacco causes metabolic and other physical changes that result in tobacco users weighing at least several pounds less than they would weigh if they did not use tobacco (e.g., Williamson et al., 1991). When they quit using tobacco, this weight returns. For most smokers, this weight is limited to 6 to 12 pounds. For some, however, the difference is as much as 30 pounds. The possibility of gaining this weight after quitting smoking can be disconcerting and discouraging, and it motivates many smokers to continue using tobacco.

Common sense would dictate that a quitting smoker could avoid weight gain by dieting while stopping smoking. This may seem to make sense, but it can be a bad strategy, as researchers have found (e.g., Hall, Tunstall, Vila, & Duffy, 1992). Those quitting smokers who tolerate weight gain and then deal with it once smoking is behind them are more successful at avoiding relapse than those who attempt to diet while quitting smoking. Those who combine quitting smoking with a moderate exercise plan, however, tend to succeed in quitting. The difference between successful ex-smokers and those who relapse is one of attitude and approach. The focus, as it turns out, must be on enjoying and encouraging health, not on straining against the scales to avoid gaining 5 or 10 pounds when trying to quit smoking.

Just One Puff?

A dieter who wants to lose weight probably can sneak an occasional piece of chocolate or a bite of cheesecake without seriously compromising his or her health. But a smoker who is quitting cannot indulge in even a single puff, because any smoking during an attempt to quit greatly increases the likelihood of a full relapse. Most smokers require between four and six serious attempts at quitting—even with therapy—before they can become permanently abstinent (Food and Drug Administration, 1995). Any single attempt to quit without behavioral treatment, medication, or other intervention, has about a 5% chance of success (Cohen et al., 1989). The addition of group therapy and behavioral treatment raises the success rate about fourfold. Also, adding nicotine replacement medicine typically doubles the rate of success compared with that produced by placebo (Hughes, in press).

Relapse may be triggered by a social situation, an unexpected stressor, or by a craving. Treatment should be designed to help smokers prepare for these relapse triggers. When attempting to quit smoking, a smoker cannot indulge in an occasional cigarette. This does not mean that the lapse represented by a single cigarette spells the ex-smoker's doom, but it does mean that even one puff of smoke puts an ex-smoker at high risk for going back to smoking.

Keep Trying Until You Succeed

It is important that the individual not become discouraged by failed attempts to quit (Kozlowski, 1987). Smokers can learn from previous attempts to quit.

They can learn not to be fooled by thinking they can smoke "just one more ciga-rette." They can learn what techniques work best for them. They can also learn to try harder the next time they try.

A Matter of Responsibility

Whose responsibility is it that a tobacco user is addicted to tobacco? Some people blame themselves for having a physical and psychological dependence on to-bacco, without recognizing that most tobacco users start with a few cigarettes when they are young, at a time of life when they are not necessarily inclined to make decisions based on long-term consequences (Russell, 1990). This self-blame can become a destructive process that keeps them from successfully quit-ting their tobacco use. Whatever the reasons for the initial use of tobacco, the fact is that tobacco is an addictive product, probably much more addictive than most first-time users imagine and comparable to so-called hard drugs in addictive prop-erties (Benowitz, 1998a; Hughes, Higgins, & Bickel, 1994). Even if the physical addiction itself is not established for weeks or even years, the psychologically re-inforcing qualities of tobacco provide powerful motivation for continuing tobacco use to the point of dependence.

It can be helpful for smokers and other tobacco users, particularly those who want to quit, to realize that most tobacco products are deliberately designed to be maximally addictive (Hoffman & Hoffman, 1997; also, see Chapters 4, 5, 6, and 7). The dose of nicotine in a cigarette is carefully controlled during its manufac-ture, and the delivery mechanism is carefully structured to provide an optimally addictive smoking experience. Cigarettes and other tobacco products are de-signed to capture the user in a web of lifelong cravings for a cigarette. This is no accident; the creation of modern tobacco products followed years of research, testing, and development by tobacco manufacturers, research that continues even today.

Tobacco manufacturers, however, are in the business of selling tobacco prod-ucts, not helping smokers quit. For help in quitting, smokers have to look else-where, primarily to health care providers, to medications, and to their own re-sources. In developed countries, such as the United States and England, the burden for helping tobacco users quit now rests on the shoulders of professionals such as physicians, dentists, psychologists, and nurses. At this point, few of these professionals have formal training in providing tobacco dependence treatment (Ferry, Grissino, & Runfola, 1999; Richmond, Debono, Larcos, & Kehoe, 1998).

The reason that national organizations such as England's Royal College of Physicians (Raw et al., 1998) and the U.S. Agency for Health Care Policy and Research (Fiore et al., 1996) have placed this responsibility on health care providers is a simple one: With help such as medications and counseling, the long-term success rates at least double and triple, and in some cases, these measures are as much as 10 times as effective as quitting without assistance (Hughes, in press). For this reason, the responsibility rests not only on the smoker but also on professionals who need to learn tools and skills that can help the smoker's chances of succeeding.

■ The Professional's Role

Health care professionals in both developed and developing countries have been charged with the responsibility of monitoring the tobacco use of their patients and clients and offering to help them quit (Fiore et al., 1996; Raw et al., 1998; World Health Organization, 1999), even if the patient has other complicating disorders (American Psychiatric Association, 1996). The guideline set by the U.S. Agency for Health Care Policy and Research (AHCPR; Fiore et al., 1996) explicitly instructs primary care clinicians (those who provide health care services for a problem other than smoking per se) to use the following strategies, regardless of whether smoking cessation is the patient's reason for coming to the clinician:

- ■ *Strategy 1: Ask*—Systematically identify all tobacco users at every visit. Implement an office-wide system that ensures that tobacco-use status is queried and documented for every patient at every clinic visit.
- ■ *Strategy 2: Advise*—Strongly urge all smokers to quit. In a clear, strong, and personalized manner, urge every smoker to quit.
- ■ *Strategy 3: Identify*—Find smokers willing to make a quit attempt. Ask every smoker if he or she is willing to attempt to quit.
- ■ *Strategy 4: Assist*—Aid the patient in quitting. Help the patient with a quit plan. Encourage nicotine replacement except in special circumstances. Give key advice on successful quitting. Provide supplementary materials.
- ■ *Strategy 5: Arrange*—Schedule follow-up contact either in person or by telephone.

The 1998 British version of these guidelines represents a comparable set of strategies. It also includes a section outlining the cost-effectiveness of smoking cessation (Parrott, Godfrey, Raw, West, & McNeill, 1998).

With help and with repeated efforts, as many as half of all smokers do eventually succeed in quitting. However, health care providers have far to go to reach the goal of providing all the help they can. Only a small minority of health insurance companies and health maintenance organizations in the United States provide coverage for treatment of nicotine dependence (see multiple reports on implementation of the AHCPR guideline, *Tobacco Control, 6,* Supplement 1). Incongruously, it is not uncommon for a health or dental insurance plan to cover the cost of treating tobacco-related disease but to fail to underwrite the far less onerous cost of preventing such disease. To their credit, some health care providers routinely inquire about tobacco-use status anyway, offering assistance even when it is not reimbursed by insurance or paid by the patient.

A key element in effective assistance for tobacco users is the training of health care professionals. This is a worldwide challenge. Only one third of the medical schools in the world instruct medical students in tobacco dependence treatment, even though 88% include tobacco as a curriculum topic (Richmond, Debono, Larcos, & Kehoe, 1998). Although this figure seems low, it is probably greater than the percentage of psychologists, social workers, and other nonmedical personnel who receive training in helping patients and clients quit using tobacco. Even in the most developed countries in Europe and the Americas, this educational undertaking is only in its early stages. Many students undertaking professional training will need to assume the responsibility themselves for learning how best to help their tobacco using patients.

At present, a range of professionals—and others with no professional training at all—offer a variety of treatment options for the treatment of tobacco dependence. An uncounted array of unproven herbal remedies; gadgets, such as earlobe rings and computerized wristwatches; and techniques are touted as ways to help tobacco users quit using tobacco. Only a limited number of approaches have been demonstrated to be successful. In general, the effectiveness of treatment reflects what is called a dose-response relationship; the more intense and long lasting the treatment, the more effective it is in facilitating long-term abstinence. Just as a higher dose of ibuprofen can help alleviate a headache not helped by a lower dose, more intense treatment for tobacco dependence can be more effective than less intense treatment (Burns, in press; Hughes, in press.)

Of course, the success of treatment depends in part on who is providing the treatment. Some persons who offer tobacco dependence treatment have little to no training specific to tobacco and have little to offer except moral support. No standards exist at present for training, although the AHCPR and the British guidelines provide a standard for delivery of treatment. An ideal situation, many researchers believe, would be for tobacco dependence training to become a certified specialty available for a wide range of health professionals and others. At this writing, specialist training is limited to programs such as that at the Mayo Clinic's Nicotine Dependence Treatment Center.

A primary question is just who would be providing certified service—only those with medical or dental training? Should this include technicians and hygienists? Pharmacists? Psychologists and other counselors? Educators? If providing treatment rests only in the realm of medical personnel, then little help will be accessible to those without easy access to medical professionals. On the other hand, can those with no medical or psychological training provide sufficient help? The early efforts toward certification programs in the United States reflect the goal of finding a balance between the need for some medical background and the need for widely accessible treatment. Small groups of professionals in most "helping" fields, such as pharmacology and nursing, are taking the lead in piloting training programs that will prepare students to take an effective role in helping patients and clients quit using tobacco (e.g., Sinclair et al., 1998). Widespread implementation of these programs is some years in the future, however.

▨ What Should Treatment Involve?

For most smokers hoping to quit, nicotine replacement is worth serious consideration. Another desirable component of treatment is person-to-person treatment of some kind, preferably delivered over four to seven sessions. Generally, treatment is more effective if it is delivered over a longer period of time, within the limits of the resources available. U.S. and British guidelines recommend that treatment for stopping smoking should include the following elements:

Problem-Solving

- Recognition of situations that will increase the risk of smoking or relapse, such as being around other smokers, being under time pressure, getting into an argument, negative moods, or using alcohol
- Developing coping skills to identify and practice problem-solving in avoiding situations with risk for relapse, learning strategies to reduce negative moods, changing lifestyle to reduce stress and produce pleasure, and learning activities that detract from urges to smoke
- Providing information about smoking and quitting, including the nature of withdrawal symptoms, addiction, and the realities of relapse

Support

■ Encouraging the smoker through explaining effective treatment methods and providing confidence in the smoker's ability to quit

■ Communicating concern by asking about the smoker's feelings and concerns, being willing to help, and being open to the smoker's fears and difficulties

■ Encouraging the smoker to discuss the process of quitting, through asking about reasons for quitting, difficulties encountered in quitting, successes, and concerns

These techniques are part of a relatively low-intensity treatment program that can be provided to some extent by most care providers over a period of weeks and months. It does not cost a great deal in time or money for a clinician to ask a patient who is quitting smoking to return for a follow-up visit, nor does it cost much time or money to call the patient on the telephone to offer support and advice. Low-intensity, low-cost interventions can be delivered to large numbers of smokers through existing routes of health care delivery, including health maintenance organizations and routine medical encounters. In conjunction with prevention programs and public health campaigns, these interventions can dramatically reduce the overall rate of tobacco use.

Some smokers, however, require more intensive treatment. This may be the case for those who are heavily dependent on tobacco and who have physical problems that require them to quit immediately. Few such programs exist, even in the best hospitals and treatment centers. Few clinicians are trained to provide such treatment, even if they are capable of working with less dependent smokers. A 1998 U.S. ad hoc advisory group reported to the Center for the Advancement of Health that "our nation currently lacks the capacity to deliver effective basic and intensive treatment to those who need it." They recommended that the top priority in allocating funds for treatment of tobacco use be "to develop the systems, competencies, and resources needed to deliver and monitor integrated, evidence-based basic and intensive treatment to tobacco users."

■ What's Wrong With This Picture?

The shortage of intensive treatment facilities underscores the lack of attention and interest that tobacco dependence treatment has received in the medical community until recent years and the urgency of providing medical service that is far less expensive than typical disease treatments. Amazingly, medical diagnostic and treatment equipment costing many millions of dollars is routinely employed at hundreds of medical centers throughout the United States, but few centers provide the relatively straightforward stop-smoking assistance that would prevent the need for expensive equipment and costly treatments. In fact, it was only in the late 1980s and the 1990s that U.S. hospitals began requiring that patients who were smokers not smoke in their rooms and that hospitals themselves became smoke-free environments.

Why the delay, when reports about the health hazards of smoking have been public for several decades? Much of the answer lies in the marketing strategy that made the Marlboro Man the "advertising icon of the century," in the elite company of the Energizer Bunny, Betty Crocker, and the Pillsbury Doughboy (*Top 10 Ad Icons,* 1999). It was only a few decades ago that some physicians endorsed cigarettes in advertising as a way to reduce anxiety, stay slim, and enhance pleasure. Since then, tobacco advertising has promoted false health benefits (e.g., filters, menthol, and "light" cigarettes) while covering the globe with powerful images associating independence and enjoyment with cigarette smoking.

The public health community, on the other hand, has had the burden of demonstrating that tobacco is dangerous to health and that quitting benefits health (USDHHS, 1988, 1990). The tobacco image is one of enjoyment; the public health message is by its nature negative and perhaps less compelling. In addition, tobacco's widespread use has lulled many people into a sense of acceptance and security about tobacco. It can't be that bad, many people assume, or it wouldn't be so popular and wouldn't be associated with positive activities such as riding horses, playing outdoors, and being sociable. After all, millions of people smoke, and if it were that bad, governments would do something—right?

Governments have done something, in countries as diverse as Canada, New Zealand, and Ghana (World Health Organization, 1999). Government funds are now being spent for researching and implementing effective prevention and treatment programs. For these and other reasons, many in the worldwide health community, as well as some insurers and health organizations, have recently begun taking the hazards of using tobacco and the need for treatment seriously.

Even so, it is still common to see something like the following notice in the "Principal Benefits and Coverages" brochure for a dental plan:

Nutritive counseling for the control of dental disease	No Charge
Oral hygiene instruction	No Charge
Tobacco counseling for the control and prevention of oral disease	Not Covered

(From PacifiCare Dental Plan 590, copyright 1997, distributed 1999)

What will change this state of affairs? Most proponents of tobacco treatment recognize that the cost-effectiveness of treatment for tobacco dependence will change the minds of those who make payment decisions (Raw et al., 1998). Preventing disease is far less costly than treating disease. For the same amount that it costs to treat one lung cancer or heart patient, dozens of smokers can be assisted in quitting.

Using Resources Creatively

Awareness and creativity can be excellent resources in making a successful attempt to quit and the best defense against relapse. Consider what recommendations you might make in these situations, if you were a specialist in treating tobacco dependence.

- *A smoker typically lights up at the same point in his commute to work every weekday morning. As he passes the same billboard each morning, he lights up a cigarette and starts to smoke. For him, this moment is one of life's small pleasures, as he mentally prepares himself for the workday ahead. After several years of following this pattern, he quits smoking but finds that just driving past this billboard triggers strong urges to smoke. What could he do? (Hint: Consider the impact of cues in the environment that can trigger a relapse.)*
- *A woman smoker with several small children enjoys getting together with friends one afternoon a week to drink coffee, smoke, and chat at a local coffee shop. The friends hire a babysitter together for this weekly respite from the demands of motherhood. This woman wants to quit smoking but fears she cannot quit without also quitting this weekly tradition. What are her options? (Hint: Social support is a critical part of quitting for good when a smoker has linked tobacco use with social settings.)*
- *An office worker takes on a part-time evening job to supplement her income. This keeps her up late several nights a week. She smokes to stay awake on the job and on the drive home. She has tried to quit smoking many times, but this time she fears that she would jeopardize her part-time work as well as her driving safety if she quits smoking. What should she do? (Hint: Nicotine replacement products can lengthen the quitting process by preventing withdrawal-associated performance degradations.)*

▶ *A high school senior has been using smokeless tobacco without his parents' knowledge for several years. He and some of his friends started using smokeless tobacco on a dare in junior high school and soon found themselves addicted. When he gets together with his friends, they still want to use tobacco. However, the young man's parents have discovered his tobacco use and have offered to help him quit. He sees no reason to quit, except to please them. What else might motivate him to quit? (Hint: He and his friends can decide to quit together; also, he can seek help.)*

▶ *An elderly man has started attending a church with strict health codes that prohibit the use of tobacco. He longs to be part of the congregation but cannot give up his cigars. Even though his clothes reek of tobacco smoke, people at church accept him and welcome him. However, he is ashamed that he cannot keep the same health standards that others seem to be following, and he confesses this to the minister, adding that he is embarrassed to come to church. If you were his minister what might you tell him? (Hint: A church where smoking is forbidden can provide a social structure free of the relapse triggers and cues he might find in other social settings.)*

▶ *An elderly neighbor is diagnosed with chronic obstructive lung disease and decides it is not worth quitting smoking, because he will probably die soon anyway. Why deny himself this small pleasure? If you were his physician, what might you tell him? (Hint: Quitting smoking at any time can improve health and can boost one's immune functioning and capacity for healing. [USDHHS, 1990])*

Summary

Cigarette smokers and users of other tobacco products need to stop using these products completely and as soon as possible. It usually takes more than one attempt for a smoker to succeed in giving up smoking. The health community needs to encourage and support smoking cessation. Standards have been developed for the treatment of tobacco use problems. These standards need to be implemented to help more and more people stop smoking.

Further Reading

Brigham, J. (1998). *Dying to quit: Why we smoke and how we stop.* Washington, DC: National Academy Press.

This provides an overview of the major issues involved in quitting smoking—addiction to tobacco, the reinforcing properties of tobacco, its affective and cognitive impact, sex differences in using and quitting tobacco, and basic principles behind treatment and relapse prevention.

Fiore, M. C., Bailey, W. C., Cohen, S. J. et al. (2000, June). *Treating tobacco use and dependence. Clinical practice guideline.* Rockville, MD: U.S. Department of Health and Human Services. (Available by telephone order, 800-358-9295; mail order, Publication Clearinghouse, P.O. Box 8547, Silver Spring, MD 20907; www.surgeongeneral.gov/tobacco/default.htm)

This is the U.S. government's official "gold standard" for treatment of tobacco dependence, a revised and updated version of the 1996 guideline that set the standard for treatment.

Piasecki, M., & Newhouse, P. A. (Eds.). (2000). *Nicotine in psychiatry: Psychopathology and emerging therapeutics.* Washington, DC: American Psychiatric Press.

This volume of edited articles provides a useful overview of the relationship between tobacco and psychiatric disorders, with an emphasis on treatment issues.

Raw, M. (2000). *Kick the habit: How to stop smoking and stay stopped.* London: BBC Worldwide.

Raw's publication, available by mail order through U.K. outlets such as www.amazon.co.uk (but at this writing not directly available in the United States) provides stop-smoking guidelines in accordance with England's official recommendations for quitting smoking. These recommendations closely parallel those made by the U.S. government (Fiore et al., 2000).

10

Tobacco, Public Health, and Policy

For a successful technology, reality must take precedence
over public relations, for Nature cannot be fooled.

—Richard Feynman, Nobel Laureate (1988)

New approaches to tobacco control policy have the potential to contribute to the creation of longer and healthier lives for millions of people; alternatively, new policies could worsen their fate. The effect will depend on the nature of the policy and how it is implemented. Designing and implementing tobacco control policies to reduce the death and disease caused by tobacco will require attention to factors as diverse as attitudes about the place of tobacco in society, the utility of cigarettes in controlling body weight, the addicting effects of tobacco-delivered nicotine, and governmental reliance on tobacco product tax revenues. Public policy is a kind of technology (see quotation above), and the intention of doing good does not ensure that good will, in reality, be done. Public policy related to tobacco must be evaluated on the basis of the effects it produces.

This chapter will describe the prominent factors that must be considered in the development of tobacco control policies intended to improve public health. A core premise is that no single policy will address all of the issues, but rather that enlightened policies and strategies will consist of an evolution of incrementally improving approaches for many years to come. In detailing what is needed in creating effective tobacco policy, our intention is to educate readers of this text so that they may notice and take advantage of the diverse opportunities they may have to shape the evolution of tobacco policy.

■ What Is Tobacco Policy?

It may be useful to begin with some discussion of what policy is and what we mean by *policy* in the context of tobacco control. *Policy* is a systematic approach to achieve a particular end result by providing goals, guidance, and specific strategies. A policy thus functions as a compass to help guide decision making and develop specific ways to implement the policy. *Tobacco control policy* refers to policy that is focused on controlling tobacco and its use so as to reduce disease.

In other areas of society, our nation has adopted policies on diverse issues ranging from policies aimed at reducing poverty to policies designed to foster better medical care to policies that address protecting wilderness areas and improving air quality. In each of these domains, the policy helps decision makers evaluate the various potential actions and strategies. For example, our national policy to improve air quality includes addressing emissions from factories, automobiles, and electricity producing facilities. Governmental agencies such as the Departments of Transportation and Energy become involved, although one agency with particular expertise, the Environmental Protection Agency, takes a lead, coordinating role. Strategies ranging from economic incentives, such as tax deductions for reducing emissions and fines for exceeding standards, to the prohibition of burning certain categories of toxins are implemented. Analogously, the abuse of addictive drug use, including tobacco, is addressed by the White House Office of National Drug Control Policy, which coordinates policies that are then developed by various other agencies of the U.S. Federal Government, including the Department of Education and the Department of Defense.

For tobacco policy, the lead role is taken by the Office on Smoking and Health of the Centers for Disease Control and Prevention in Atlanta, Georgia, and by the U.S. surgeon general. Virtually every other department of government then works to develop its own polices and strategies of implementation in an effort to be consistent with the nationally espoused strategy. This does not mean that all federal government efforts concerning tobacco are perfectly consistent and coordinated, or that every other department has the same priorities as the Office on Smoking and Health and the surgeon general; however, the general policy does provide guidance and consideration for other departments in their own strategic planning and day-to-day affairs. For example, the Office of National Drug Control Policy generally places its emphasis on illicit drugs of abuse, but it works with the Office on Smoking and Health to address concerns from both offices regarding the harm associated with tobacco use and the involvement of tobacco in other drug abuse.

Policies become real through strategies. Policies become real and can change society when specific enabling strategies are implemented. For example, the elimination of lead from automobile fuel to reduce toxin emissions, urine testing of military personnel for illicit drugs to discourage drug abuse, and workplace smoking restrictions to reduce environmental smoke exposure to nonsmokers are all examples of specific strategies that support a broader policy goal. The development and implementation of specific strategies is often more difficult than the development of the general policy. For example, most people would probably support goals to improve air quality, decrease illicit drug abuse, and reduce smoking prevalence. However, improving air quality by closing factories, reducing drug abuse by mass urine testing, and decreasing smoking prevalence by raising cigarette taxes are all strategies that generate controversy. Some objection to such strategies comes from affected industries and individuals, but regardless of the source of opposition and voice of controversy, the implementation of policies through specific strategies can be constrained by political, business, and constitutional considerations.

Policies and strategies can have unintended consequences. Well-intended policies and strategies can lead to adverse unintended consequences. For example, the strategy of mandating collision-activated airbags in automobiles in the 1990s had the general and intended effect of reducing major injuries in automobile accidents. An unintended effect, however, was that some children and small adults were seriously injured or killed by the explosive deployment of the airbag itself in some minor collisions that would have been unlikely to have caused serious injury had the person been secured only by a standard shoulder restraint system and had the airbag not been deployed. Reviews of automobile accident data and the operation of the systems helped to identify the problem (overly forceful deployment specifications based on the needs of average-size male adults). Corrective actions were then taken to maximize the benefits for most people while minimizing the risks for the vulnerable. Specifically, strategies included providing warnings about seating small people in the front seat of the automobile and installing switches so that the airbag system could be turned off for small persons. Strategies for reducing the risk of injury in automobiles, detecting unintended consequences, and continuing to refine the strategies are ongoing and have contributed to a dramatic decline in deaths per traveled mile in the United States over the past several decades; but the process is continually evolving, adapting to changing challenges, new technological opportunities, and ever increasing standards for safety.

Similarly, strategies to control tobacco use can backfire. Just as there is a term for unintended disorders caused by physicians (*iatrogenic*), a term has been proposed for disorders caused by those trying to do good (*eupraxigenic*; Kozlowski, 2000). Although some public education efforts about the harms of smoking have likely contributed to the dramatic declines in the prevalence of smoking, some school-based smoking prevention programs have been demonstrated scientifically to be ineffective, yet they can continue to occupy valuable space in the curriculum and give parents and the community a false sense that they are doing something productive to stop tobacco use by children (Kozlowski, Coambs, Ferrence, & Adlaf, 1989). The need for public relations efforts requires that there be prevention programs in the schools; yet science should be employed to ensure that these programs actually work. The tragedy of the low-tar cigarette is another example of a policy that produced results that were unintended by the public health community (see Chapter 8).

Unintended consequences of policies and strategies are to be expected, but in general can be minimized by analyses prior to the launch of new approaches and by postlaunch surveillance to detect the consequences and to enable corrective actions. For example, continuous air quality monitoring can quickly detect if a change in a manufacturing technology has introduced a known toxin into the air. In the case of the Federal Trade Commission's efforts to stimulate the use of lower-toxin cigarettes, no specific surveillance system was put in place to determine if these cigarettes reduced the motivation to quit or to determine if new cigarette designs actually resulted in smokers obtaining high levels of nicotine and tar or if these cigarettes might have contributed to a different type of lung cancer (see Chapter 8).

▨ Tobacco Policy Background: The Driving Force

Today, tobacco policy is developing alongside issues such as global warming, health care, and international treaties governing trade and landmines. These issues are being raised by agencies and organizations including the U.S. Congress, the European Union, and the World Health Organization. The issues under consideration by these and other public policy-making bodies include the nicotine dosing capacity of cigarettes, the social and physiological needs for tobacco, as well as taxation rates, and international trade approaches. Biobehavioral issues are in the forefront, because they determine whether or not policies will be successful. What has driven such a major and pervasive reevaluation of tobacco control policy?

The driving force for these efforts is the grim reality that smoking-attributable deaths are accelerating globally and are projected to exceed all other forms of preventable premature death early in the 21st century. In the United States, the current projections of smoking-attributable death and disease illustrate the need for improved policy and suggest ways that policy might be improved. As shown in Figure 10.1, the annual mortality rate attributable to cigarette smoking was about 400,000 per year throughout the 1990s and was not expected to change drastically without revolutionary advances in the treatment and prevention of tobacco-caused diseases. Thus, as indicated by Figure 10.1, more than 20 million people who were smoking in the year 2000 could die prematurely of smoking-attributable diseases within the first few decades of the 21st century. This accumulation of tobacco-attributable mortality will likely continue as long as the pipeline of smokers continues to be fed by new smokers and as long as most smokers continue to smoke for several decades.

Three Potential Trajectories for Cumulative Tobacco-Caused Deaths in America

Although smoking-attributable diseases do occur in young smokers, the skyrocketing mortality rates begin largely with smokers who have smoked for several decades and are approaching the age of 50 (Burns, Benowitz, et al., 1997). Thus, as shown in Figure 10.1, if strategies to prevent the onset of smoking become dramatically more effective, the benefit, with respect to the reduction of premature deaths, might not be clearly evidenced for approximately 30 years, during which time many millions more smokers would die prematurely.

On the other hand, reducing the extent and prevalence of tobacco toxin exposure and stimulating and supporting cessation efforts could have substantial bene-

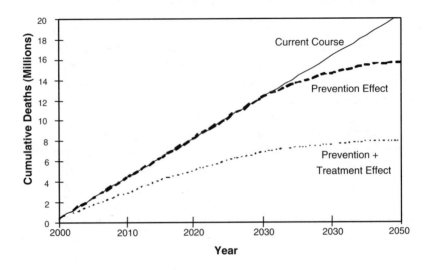

Figure 10.1. Projection of Tobacco-Caused Mortality Based on Present Trends ("Current Course") Compared With Projections of No New Smokers ("Prevention Effect") and Projections in Which Smoking Is Reduced by Both Prevention and Smoking Treatment Efforts ("Prevention + Treatment Effects")
SOURCE: Henningfield and Slade (1998).

fits within a few years (Henningfield & Slade, 1998; Shiffman et al., 1997). This is because many adverse effects of tobacco, such as increased risk of heart disease, can be reduced within months of cessation (Chapter 9; Henningfield & Slade, 1998). The combination of increased treatment accessibility, effective means of reducing tobacco consumption, and prevention of new initiation could sharply reduce tobacco-related deaths within a few years and could prevent millions of deaths within a few decades. Thus, the greatest overall benefit to public health would be produced by policies that lead to both increased rates of cessation among established smokers and diminished rates of smoking uptake by nonsmokers. Unfortunately, efforts to prevent smoking by youth historically have garnered substantially more support and emphasis than efforts to support treatment among adults and youth who already use tobacco. There needs to be a balanced approach to prevention and treatment.

▧ Policy Goals

As evidenced in the historic tobacco policy debates in the U.S. Congress in the late 1990s, the goals of the participants were as varied as the participants themselves (Hilts, 1998; Kessler, 2000). The tobacco industry favored policy that would restore their legitimacy as a business enterprise, protect their current and future marketing opportunities, and obtain shelter from litigation. Health advocates wanted virtually the opposite of everything sought by the tobacco industry, with the assumption that the only way to reduce death and disease would be to greatly curtail the ability of the industry to market tobacco products. Scientists wanted a more stable research enterprise dedicated to better understanding, preventing, and treating tobacco addiction and its disease consequences. Pharmaceutical companies and other corporations that sold treatment products wanted incentives for developing and marketing treatments for tobacco dependence. State attorneys general sought fiscal relief for the medical costs of their citizens and assurance of fewer tobacco-caused diseases in the future.

Cutting across virtually all boundaries, however, was general agreement on the importance of reducing the death and disease caused by tobacco products. Even the tobacco industry, while denying in courts of law that specific causal connections linked tobacco product use and premature mortality, began to pursue strategies that it claimed could lessen the risk of smoking-attributable diseases (e.g., Schwartz, 1999). The disease reduction goal was a hallmark of the 1964 U.S. surgeon general's report and was the most important consideration when the Food and Drug Administration first proposed its tobacco rule in 1995.

▧ Tobacco Policy in the United States

Because the official determination by the U.S. surgeon general in 1964 indicated that cigarette smoking was a major preventable cause of death and disease, the U.S. Government has stated a core health policy goal of reducing smoking-related disease. Strategies include those intended to prevent initiation of use in young people, increase the cessation efforts in established smokers, and reduce the toxicity of cigarettes for continuing smokers. At first blush, these may seem like straightforward and readily achievable strategies. If the United States could rally to reduce the spread and consequences of HIV, eradicate smallpox and polio, and put a man on the moon, it could surely act to thwart the cause of 20% of all deaths in the United States. Unfortunately, however, tobacco seems to have been a more challenging problem than any of the foregoing examples; four decades following the release of the 1964 surgeon general's report, tobacco continues to account for approximately 20% of all premature mortalities in the United States, with no dramatic reduction in sight. What happened? What went wrong? Did anything go right?

Following the findings of the 1964 surgeon general's report and the findings of subsequent surgeons general's reports, various governmental agencies and departments developed separate policies and strategies for supporting the broad policy of reducing tobacco use and disease. The U.S. Congress required health warning labels on cigarettes packages. The Department of Education integrated tobacco prevention programs into school curricula. The Department of Defense restricted tobacco use by recruits and offered cessation treatment for military personnel who smoked. The National Institutes of Health supported research on the health effects of tobacco and the treatment of nicotine addiction. Overall, smoking prevalence declined from nearly 40% in the 1960s to about 25% in the year 2000, and awareness that smoking was harmful increased.

Some policies were more effective than others, however. For example, research from the National Institutes of Health enormously expanded the knowledge base and contributed to better communications about the harms of smoking, the benefits of quitting, and how to quit. The National Cancer Institute reviewed state and local legislative efforts in the United States (National Cancer Institute [NCI], 2000). The approval of smoking cessation medications for over-the-counter sales provided consumers with easier access to effective cessation aids and was accompanied by increased utilization of treatment (Centers for Disease Control and Prevention [CDC], 2000).

On the other hand, some efforts were countered and even neutralized by creative strategies employed by the tobacco industry. Marketing campaigns targeting children resulted in a higher level of recognition of cigarette company icons such as RJ Reynolds's Joe Camel in the 1990s than that of Mickey Mouse (Fischer, Schwartz, Richard, Goldstein, & Rojas, 1991). The sponsorship of auto racing, tennis, and other sports and cultural activities garnered more actual exposure of cigarette brand logos (on cars, baseball fences, and in the names of events) than occurred prior to the prohibition of television advertising. Perhaps one of the biggest failures was the Federal Trade Commission's (FTC) effort to spur the use and development of less toxic cigarettes by requiring that cigarettes be measured for tar and nicotine delivery levels according to a protocol developed jointly by the FTC and the tobacco industry (Chapter 8). By designing cigarettes that would test low on smoking machines and then using these ratings to support advertising, brand names, and marketing efforts invoking labels such as *light* and *low tar,* the tobacco industry turned this public health strategy into a marketing tool. In fact, a major unintended consequence, from a public health perspective, was that the tobacco industry was able to market cigarettes that would delay the quitting process and would provide an alternative to quitting (Kozlowski & O'Connor, 2000). What enabled this unintended consequence to persist, in part, was the lack of oversight by an agency with experience in drug-dosing issues, such as the Food and Drug Administration.

Policy Efforts in the 1990s

The 1990s were a turning point for tobacco policy development. Congressman Henry Waxman held historic hearings on tobacco product health effects and marketing in 1994 (Committee on Energy and Commerce, 1995). These hearings yielded one of the most galvanizing photos of the decade. It showed tobacco industry senior executives raising their right hands to take an oath before testifying that their products were not addictive and did not cause cancer. This led to congressional review of specific strategies including the imposition of substantially increased taxes on cigarettes, support for FDA regulation of tobacco products, and recognition of the shortcomings of the FTC approach to cigarette tar and nicotine ratings. The tobacco industry resisted with an incredible display of lobbying force in Washington, DC. Although it had previously asserted that nicotine was only an incidental element of tobacco that contributed to the sensory pleasures of smoking, it now screamed that policies such as these would be tantamount to cigarette prohibition and would lead to major criminal and smuggling activity (Committee on Energy and Commerce, 1988, 1995).

On August 23, 1996, the President of the United States and the Commissioner of the Food and Drug Administration announced that cigarettes and smokeless tobacco would join the foods and medicines regulated by the FDA. The purpose of the FDA rule was to reduce the death and disease caused by tobacco use by reducing the access and appeal of tobacco among children and adolescents (Kessler et al., 1996). The first wave of implementation of that jurisdiction became effective on February 28, 1997. Additional regulations were then phased in over the next several years, with limitations imposed by court challenges from the tobacco industry. Ultimately, the Supreme Court ruled in the spring of 2000 that despite the enormity of the health problem and the probable need for jurisdiction, such authority ran counter to the intent of Congress in establishing the FDA, and

Congress therefore would need to pass legislation granting such jurisdiction (Kessler, 2000, 2001).

At about the same time that the FDA issued its 1996 Final Rule, in which it asserted jurisdiction over cigarettes and smokeless tobacco, an increasing number of states filed lawsuits against the tobacco industry (Hilts, 1998; Kessler et al., 1996). The lawsuits adopted variations of the legal theory that because the tobacco industry had knowingly marketed products that caused addiction and harm and did not act to reduce the toxic and addictive effects it could be held liable for the health consequences of cigarettes. A core premise of the lawsuits was that the tobacco industry was liable for a portion of the medical expenses paid by the states to treat persons made ill by the use of tobacco products because the toxic and addictive effects of cigarettes had been willfully manipulated by the manufacturers, and knowledge that could have lead to enlightened tobacco control policies had been suppressed (Hilts, 1998).

Due in part to these regulatory and legal activities, the public release of previously secret documents from tobacco companies and their law firms grew from a trickle to a flood during the 1990s, adding further fuel to the fires of regulators and potential litigants against the tobacco industry (Hirschhorn, 2000; Hurt & Robertson, 1998; Slade et al., 1995). These public disclosures and litigation efforts drove major U.S. tobacco companies and several state attorneys general in 1997 to develop a proposed resolution in which the states would drop their lawsuits in exchange for nearly $400 billion in payments from the tobacco industry and an industry agreement to reduce marketing practices targeted toward children. Many of the objectives of the resolution were commented on and discussed in various scientific journals as well as in the mainstream press (Burns, Benowitz, et al., 1997; Douglas, 1998; Henningfield, 1997). However, such an agreement required ratification by the U.S. Congress. From the outset, it was clear that Congress would not simply adopt a resolution offered by the industry and several state attorneys general. It was also clear that representatives with a wide range of potential interests would lobby for legislation to serve their ends. Remarkably, legislation did get to the floor of Congress with enough votes to pass. However, the legislation did not have enough supporters to override a procedural issue that opponents invoked to kill the legislation. The legislation died in the summer of 1998 (Schwartz, 1999).

Despite the death of the proposed tobacco legislation, the forces that made such legislation possible continued to operate, most notably through FDA regulatory actions and increased efforts by various states to take legislation into their own hands. For example, the state of Massachusetts required disclosure of actual nicotine content information on many cigarette brands in 1998 (Henningfield,

2000). Moreover, many state governments, health care providers, and citizens launched a flurry of lawsuits in the vacuum left by the absence of comprehensive legislation. The one certainty that emerged was that status quo tobacco policies would not be sustained. Through some combination of legal, regulatory, and legislative action, tobacco manufacturing and marketing would be forced to change in unprecedented ways (Gladwell, 2000; Kessler, 1999, 2000; Page, 1998).

Policy Challenges

Recognition of Tobacco Use as a Biobehavioral Phenomenon

We now understand tobacco use as a biobehaviorally mediated behavior involving factors including social pressures, individual desires, genetically conferred vulnerabilities, the pharmacological utility of nicotine, and the development of tolerance and dependence on nicotine. This expanded understanding has profound implications for public health, regulation, and policy. In fact, policy is the rubber of the wheels where the biobehavioral "automobile" hits the road. Perhaps nowhere is this better illustrated than by former FDA Commissioner David A. Kessler's testimony before the U.S. Congress concerning the FDA's consideration of regulating tobacco products as drugs. On March 25, 1994, he stated:

> Clearly, the possibility of FDA exerting jurisdiction over cigarettes raises many broader social issues for Congress to contemplate. It could lead to the possible removal of nicotine-containing cigarettes from the market, the limiting of the amount of nicotine in cigarettes to levels that are not addictive, or restrict access to them, unless the industry could show that nicotine-containing cigarettes are safe and effective. If nicotine were removed precipitously, millions of Americans would experience addiction withdrawal. Of course, a black market in cigarettes could develop. (Committee on Energy and Commerce, 1995)

Thus, as suggested by Kessler, simply attempting to ban cigarettes or restrict the nicotine in cigarettes could lead to problems created by the deprivation of nicotine. This is not to say that increased restrictions on cigarettes and the eventual elimination of nicotine in cigarettes were ruled out. However, as explained in a report of the American Medical Association on reducing the addictiveness of cigarettes, such actions need to be done in the context of a broad range of coordinated efforts, including those furthering increased education, substantially expanding treatment services, and increasing access to safer forms of nicotine, for those who need long-term nicotine administration (Henningfield et al., 1998). Many of the recommendations of the American Medical Association report stemmed from the concept that tobacco use is a complex, biobehaviorally mediated behavior.

Who Will Control the Nicotine?

As might be surmised from the foregoing discussion, the effects of nicotine and its role in tobacco use have made issues concerning the regulation, control, and provision of nicotine central to many tobacco control policy efforts. For example, nicotine was also central to the proposition that the FDA could regulate tobacco products; if the FDA showed that nicotine in tobacco products was having drug effects on users, then its case for regulation of tobacco products was strengthened. Although the tobacco industry fought vigorously against FDA regulation of tobacco products, the industry understood this issue well. For example, a senior researcher for Philip Morris, William Dunn, who was nicknamed the "nicotine kid" in the company, wrote a memo to his director in 1969, in which he expressed the following opinion: "I would be cautious in using the pharmaco-medical model. Do we really want to tout cigarette smoke as a drug? It is, of course, but there are dangerous FDA implications to having such conceptualization go beyond these walls" (Hurt & Robertson, 1998, p. 1176).

Historically the tobacco industry had controlled the nicotine in its products with little apparent concern for consumers' health and with extensive efforts to maximize addiction. All of this occurred with little meaningful oversight from any agency that had expertise or regulatory authority over drug delivery systems. In contrast, the safest forms of nicotine delivery, which could be lifesaving (such as the nicotine gum and patches used in treatment) were stringently regulated (Kozlowski, Appel, Frecker, & Khouw, 1982; Sweanor, 2000). This approach perpetuated an environment in which the most addictive and toxic forms of nicotine were the least regulated and were the most attractive and accessible to consumers. A core challenge to be overcome was summarized as follows in the proceedings of a conference on novel tobacco-control strategies:

> From a public health perspective, achieving the deceptively simple goal of "leveling the competitive playing field" between tobacco and treatment products would be enormously beneficial. In reality, however, making treatment for tobacco dependence as acceptable and accessible as tobacco products is fraught with obstacles. Tobacco products are designed, packaged, marketed and advertised to maximize their appeal, to increase consumption by users, to sustain users

as long as possible, to increase the chances of relapse in people who do quit, and to promote initiation in nonusers. In contrast, FDA-approved medications must be designed, marketed and advertised in ways that minimize any use beyond that for approved indications (which at present is limited to smoking cessation). (Henningfield & Slade, 1998, p. 112)

Particularly worrisome to the tobacco industry was the possibility that nicotine eventually might be prohibited from cigarettes, as proposed by Benowitz and Henningfield in 1994. In their article, Benowitz and Henningfield proposed the gradual removal of nicotine from cigarettes until the level of nicotine could no longer sustain addiction. Four years later, the American Medical Association recommended consideration of a similar proposal (Henningfield et al., 1998). Although this proposal was never acted upon by the FDA, it highlighted the need for comprehensive tobacco control policies that would address issues from the biobehavioral to the political. It should be noted that some public health experts do not support the proposal to gradually reduce the nicotine in cigarettes (e.g., Royal College of Physicians, 2000).

To the tobacco industry, which regarded nicotine as the *sine qua non* of smoking, giving up any degree of control over nicotine in tobacco products was not acceptable (FDA, 1996; Hurt & Robertson, 1998). The status quo, however, does not make sense from a public health perspective: The most contaminated and addictive forms of nicotine delivery are regulated the most leniently and are the most readily available, while the purest, safest, most highly regulated forms (treatment medicines) are more difficult to obtain. Reversing this situation will not be easy in the face of powerful opposition from the tobacco industry.

Although there has been little progress in rationally regulating tobacco products, it seems to be possible for public health groups to directly "counter-market" low-tar cigarettes (Kozlowski, Goldberg et al., 1999). Counter-marketing involves systematic opposition to the marketing of low-tar cigarettes by means of public education campaigns. There is evidence that such efforts can be successful. With extensive television advertising, the Massachusetts Department of Public Health has been able to inform smokers that light cigarettes are not better for their health, and this appears to have encouraged smokers in Massachusetts to quit smoking (Kozlowski, Yost, Stine, & Celebucki, 2000).

Coordination of Prevention and Cessation Efforts

One of the lead architects of tobacco control policy of the 20th century, former Surgeon General C. Everett Koop, kept his focus on the death and disease caused by tobacco and on the importance of comprehensive and coordinated efforts to reduce the ravages of tobacco use. For example, when some were advocating focusing tobacco control efforts on children at the expense of treating addicted smokers, Koop countered by emphasizing the importance of the big picture from a policy perspective, as in this following editorial published in the *Washington Post* in 1998:

> We must not focus our efforts so narrowly on preventing tobacco use by youth that we send smokers the message that we have abandoned them—that their addiction is their own fault and that we don't care about them. . . . There is an alternative. We can combine tobacco prevention initiatives with efforts to ensure that those who are hooked can obtain effective treatments. . . . Legitimate concern for the health of tobacco users should balance efforts to reduce the toxicity of tobacco products with the means to expedite the development of new treatments for those who are addicted. . . . Nevertheless, much remains to be done if our nation is to make tobacco dependence treatment as acceptable and readily available as tobacco itself. (Koop, 1998, p. C7)

In this statement, Koop embraced the importance of efforts to prevent and treat tobacco addiction, along with efforts to regulate the tobacco products themselves more effectively. A hallmark of Koop's conclusions is that they were consistent with the best available science. For example, a variety of lines of evidence had demonstrated that prevention and cessation efforts succeed most often when implemented together. A clear example of this was given in a study by Farkas and colleagues (1999), which showed that when parents quit smoking, their children are only half as likely to start smoking as are the children of parents who continue smoking. Moreover, the children of smoking parents are twice as likely to try to quit smoking if their parents quit (Farkas, Distefan, Choi, Gilpin, & Pierce, 1999).

One important component of a national cessation treatment infrastructure is the medicines used to support cessation. It was not until 1996 that medicines effective for helping people quit smoking could be obtained without a prescription. Even then, they were not practically accessible to the vast majority of those in need, namely lower-income cigarette smokers without the means to purchase the medications. In part, this occurred because the medications were packaged in quantities to provide seven days or more of treatment, as a way to discourage casual use by persons not committed to quitting smoking. Moreover, most health insurers and health care maintenance organizations either do not provide reimbursement for tobacco dependence treatment products or attach such stringent conditions upon reimbursement that relatively few smokers utilize the benefits

(Henningfield, 2000). Thus, in the United States, as in much of the world, it has been easy to obtain disease-causing tobacco products, and difficult to secure life-saving medicines and treatment (Koop, 1998). The foregoing situation is not unique to tobacco. In most major cities of the United States, a heroin or cocaine user could quickly get an illicit drug fix for little more than the price of a six-pack of beer, but might have to wait months to get accepted into a drug treatment clinic or methadone treatment program.

Integration of Tobacco Policy With Other Addictive Drug Policy

Although tobacco policy in the United States is largely developed by the Office on Smoking and Health, and regulations regarding illicit drug use are developed by the Office of National Drug Control Policy, the two offices do coordinate their efforts. This has followed recognition of the concept that addiction to tobacco and other addictive drugs share many biobehavioral features in common and that interactions must be considered. For example, tobacco use is a risk factor for other drug abuse (Chapter 7). In the past, policies for tobacco and other addictive drugs were conflicting and contradictory. For example, some school-based programs emphasized the dangers of illicit drugs while discounting the dangers of smoking or even providing students with smoking rooms. Many drug abuse treatment programs paid little or no attention to cigarette smoking while emphasizing the importance of a "drug-free" lifestyle.

Today this is changing, as drug abuse awareness programs for young people now increasingly include tobacco among drugs of concern and as drug abuse and alcohol treatment clinics are beginning to address tobacco among other addictions (Kozlowski, Coambs, Ferrence, & Adlaf, 1989; Kozlowski, Skinner, Kent, & Pope, 1989). This is not to imply, however, that tobacco policy should be the same as heroin policy, any more than cocaine policy should be the same as alcohol policy. As discussed in depth by one of the leading drug abuse researchers and theoreticians, Dr. Avram Goldstein (1994), similarities among addictive drugs warrant some general similarities in policies, while differences across drugs must be considered for the policies to be rational, workable, and effective. These similarities and differences include appreciation of biobehavioral effects.

Most addictive drugs are capable of modulating mood to some extent, and most have the potential to produce effects in the brain that will lead at least some users to persist in use, even in the face of harm. However, not all addictive drugs produce similar levels of intoxication, euphoria, and pain relief. Addictive drugs also vary widely in the extent and nature of damage caused to users and nonusers alike. For example, intoxication is a major side effect of alcohol consumption. Even though most alcohol users do not become dependent on or abuse alcohol, and alcohol is accepted as a licit drug, the consequences for driving while intoxicated are becoming increasingly harsh. Drugs also vary widely in their legal status, with heroin having no licit place in medicine in the United States, whereas morphine is a widely prescribed analgesic. Alcohol requires an age of procurement of 21 in most states and allows sales from licensed dealers only. Tobacco can be sold to persons 18 years and older at nearly any convenience store. Caffeine provides still another point of contrast. Caffeine is a drug with some dependence-producing qualities, but uncontrollable use of caffeine in the face of harm is relatively rare, and caffeine-attributable disease is apparently very low. Consequently, the regulatory controls over caffeine are relatively lax.

Cigarettes are smoked by more than 50 million adults in the United States, and tens of millions use other forms of tobacco. These numbers and the thorough integration of tobacco use in American culture, history, economics, and politics, must be considered in tobacco policy development. The figures set tobacco apart in many respects from illicit addictive drugs. Tobacco use is not generally associated with intoxication, and driving while smoking is not a criminal offense. In fact, the potential performance disruption caused by tobacco deprivation is increasingly considered in the implementation of smoke-free workplace policies. Moreover, tobacco farming is an important agricultural crop that provides a way of life for many people who must be considered in the development of tobacco policies. It is important, however, to appreciate that tobacco farmers are producing a *drug* crop, not a *food* crop, and that other, substitute *food* crops are unlikely to be as profitable as a *drug* crop. Other aspects of tobacco and nicotine pharmacology should be considered in the development of coordinated policies covering tobacco and other addictive drugs. The main conclusion on this point is simple: Tobacco policy should be integrated with other drug abuse policy, although differences among addictive drugs must be considered.

Regulation of Marketing

Beyond the issue of regulating nicotine itself is the regulation of tobacco product marketing in general. This is exceedingly complex, because by the mid to late 20th century, tobacco products were among the most widely and readily available of all consumer goods and were effectively sheltered from the regulations and legal remedies that made food products safer and air cleaner and that kept children from easily purchasing alcoholic beverages. For example, tobacco products were exempted from the requirements mandating meaningful content labels on potato chips, beer, and other consumable products. Tobacco products were exempted from safety regulations that reduced the unnecessary fire-starting potential of products ranging from electric lamps to pajamas; consequently, tobacco contributes to more residential fire deaths than any other product on the market (Chapman, 1999). The majority of adolescents reported that it was "easy" to obtain cigarettes and smokeless tobacco (CDC, 1996a). A package of smokeless tobacco or cigarettes could be obtained for the price of two or three soft drinks, and "kiddie" packs of five cigarettes or even single cigarettes were available in many convenience stores. Expensive packs of five cigarettes might, in contrast, help reduce smoking by adults (Kozlowski, 1986).

These conditions exist because tobacco products are not only licit but are sheltered from the ordinary regulations that protect the public from most other deadly or defective consumer products. To understand the challenges of formulating tobacco control policy, it is useful to think of tobacco products as consumer products, albeit highly toxic and addictive consumer products, and to see tobacco companies as extraordinarily effective, albeit unethical, consumer product marketers. It is also important to understand these consumer product-oriented issues, because the overall impact of any given product on its users, and on society at large, depends both on the conditions under which it is marketed and on its permitted use. This concept is fundamental, whether the product is analgesic medications, automobiles, or food.

The modern cigarette emerged at a time at the end of the 19th century when consumer product marketing approaches were different than today's approaches. Then, tobacco was often considered as basic a commodity as sugar or flour, and in times of war, as basic as armaments. The consumer product marketing philosophy of the 19th century assumed that the road to success was based primarily on finding people with a potential interest in a product or category of product and then attempting to sell them the product, based on claims of superiority or lower cost. For example, the New Shovel Company might try to convince farmers that their Dig-It-Faster shovel was the best brand to buy when someone needed a new shovel. The 20th century marketing philosophy, however, was to convince people with no real need for shovels that their tool sheds would not be complete without a shovel for emergencies, and that this shovel should be the Dig-It-Faster shovel.

Some such campaigns—such as enticing women to achieve impossible, if not outright unhealthy, body shapes—are a destructive effort to sell a wide variety of products. Efforts to increase the demand for alcoholic beverages, particularly in young people, are another example of demand marketing gone awry. However, no example is as egregious in its application or consequences as tobacco marketing. James Bonsack invented a machine that could mass-produce cigarettes. In fact, it was so fast that it could supply more cigarettes than were demanded by the market, and so the Allen and Gintner Cigarette Company of Richmond, Virginia, which owned the rights to the machine, leased it in the 1880s at a discounted rate to James Duke of Durham, North Carolina. Duke's ability to maintain his profit margin and his innovative marketing efforts contributed to an enormous market expansion in the United States and abroad that eventually led to the establishment of the British American and American Tobacco Company, which contributed to the continued expansion of the cigarette market (Cox, 2000; Slade, 1993).

Employing a market-expanding approach in selling tobacco also gave tobacco companies the advantage of addicting users while they were young and thus frequently securing them for life. One measure of the effectiveness of this strategy was that by the end of the 20th century, cigarette brands with only a few percent of the cigarette market in the United States had become highly profitable multibillion-dollar revenue streams. This marketing philosophy did not eliminate the competitive interest of different tobacco companies in fighting for their share of the market, but it did add a common interest in expanding the total market. This interest was the genesis of many shelters from regulation that protected tobacco products at the expense of consumers. It made tobacco products unique in a world in which legal, regulatory, and ordinary marketing forces governing most other areas of consumer products placed a premium on safety and benefit.

Coordination of Policies

Coordination of policies and strategies is a major challenge to policy developers. With respect to tobacco, little coordination has been evident across federal, state, and local agencies. This has led to a patchwork of inconsistent policies. Federal agencies provide financial support of tobacco farming and exports and simultaneously prohibit tobacco advertising on television. The inconsistencies have continued at the global level as well, with the World Bank helping emerging countries to develop thriving tobacco industries through financial support policies while the World Health Organization labors to reduce the spread of tobacco use through educational outreach policies. Only recently has the World Bank contributed to tobacco control efforts. Competition even occurs among public health professionals who agree with each other on core aspects of a policy but who disagree about whether to expend major resources to support treatment or to support efforts to prevent young people from initiating smoking.

Tobacco Policy in the 21st Century

Tobacco policies and regulations have the potential to provide enormous public health benefits in the 21st century in the United States and throughout the world. As mentioned earlier, the range of policy options is broad, and there are many different organizations considering tobacco policy development or refinement. These include expert committees of the World Health Organization (*Tobacco Control,* June, 2000), the United Kingdom (Royal College of Physicians, 2000), and other groups (Burns et al., 1997). Increasingly, policy discussions include consideration of biobehavioral variables, whether the issue is the importance of nicotine dependence as a consideration for tobacco taxation or potential FDA regulation given nicotine's weight-suppressing effects.

Tobacco policy needs to develop out of an awareness that nicotine is an addictive drug (Heishman, Kozlowski, & Henningfield, 1997). As should be clear, the development and implementation of strategies for tobacco control may be even more challenging than developing the guiding policies, because of the enormous range of practical, political, and economic challenges that must be confronted. The justification for considering new policy options, however, is increasingly compelling. As the Director General of the World Health Organization has observed: "The impact of actions to control tobacco [is] still not commensurate with the overall health and economic impact of tobacco use. The critical question then, is why?" (Bruntland, 2000, p. 750). As the avoidable death toll caused by unmitigated use of the most deadly forms of nicotine continues to rise, the potential impact of policy options could be among the defining characteristics of the 21st century.

Further Reading

Ferrence, R., Slade, J., Room, R., & Pope, M. (Eds.). (2000). *Nicotine and public health.* Washington, DC: American Public Health Association.

This book is based on an international conference held in Toronto in 1997 to address the health, science, and policy issues pertaining to strategies intended to reduce the harm caused by tobacco use.

Henningfield, J. E., Benowitz, N. L., Slade, J., Houston, T., Davis, R. M., & Deitchman, S. D. (1998). Reducing the addictiveness of cigarettes. *Tobacco Control, 7,* 281-293.

This paper was prepared for the American Medical Association and adopted as official AMA policy in 1998 as the basis for a policy that would reduce the prevalence of tobacco dependence by gradually reducing the nicotine permitted in commercially marketed cigarettes.

Kessler, D. (2001). *A question of intent: The great American battle with a deadly industry.* New York, NY: PublicAffairs.

The Conference on Tobacco Dependence. (1998). Innovative regulatory approaches to reduce death and disease [special issue]. *Food and Drug Law Journal, 53* (Suppl.), 1-137.

The authors and discussants included a broad range of science, policy, and regulatory experts who addressed the regulatory realities of the various proposals from the perspectives of federal agencies such as the Food and Drug Administration and the Federal Trade Commission.

References

Adler, N. E., Boyce, T., Chesney, M. A., Cohen, S., Folkman, S., Kahn, R. L., & Syme, S. L. (1994). Socioeconomic status and health: The challenge of the gradient. *American Psychologist, 49,* 15-24.

Adler, N. E., Olincy, A., Waldo, M., Harris, J. G., Griffith, J., Stevens, K., Flach, K., Nagamoto, H., Bickford, P., Leonard, S., & Freedman, R. (1998). Schizophrenia, sensory gating, and nicotinic receptors. *Schizophrenia Bulletin, 24,* 189-202.

American Council on Science and Health. (1997). *Cigarettes: What the warning label doesn't tell you.* New York: Prometheus.

American Psychiatric Association. (1980). *Diagnostic and statistical manual of mental disorders* (3rd ed.). Washington, DC: Author.

American Psychiatric Association. (1987). *Diagnostic and statistical manual of mental disorders* (3rd ed., rev.). Washington, DC: Author.

American Psychiatric Association. (1994). *Diagnostic and statistical manual of mental disorders* (4th ed.). Washington, DC: Author.

American Psychiatric Association. (1996). *Practice guideline for the treatment of patients with nicotine dependence.* Washington, DC: Author.

Austin, G. A. (1978). *Perspectives on the history of psychoactive substance use.* Rockville, MD: National Institute on Drug Abuse.

Bain, J. (1896). *Tobacco in song & story.* New York: H. M. Caldwell.

Baker, F., Ainsworth, S. R., Dye, J. T., Crammer, C., Thun, M. J., Hoffman, D., Repace, J. L., Henningfield, J. E., Slade, J., Pinney, J., Shanks, T., Burns, D. M., Connolly, G. N., & Shopland, D. R. (2000). Health risks associated with cigar smoking. *Journal of the American Medical Association, 284,* 735-740.

Balbach, E. D., & Glantz, S. A. (1995). Tobacco information in two grade school newsweeklies: A content analysis. *American Journal of Public Health, 85,* 1650-1653.

Balfour, D. J. K., & Fagerstrom, K. O. (1996). Pharmacology of nicotine and its therapeutic use in smoking cessation and neurodegenerative disorders. *Pharmacology and Therapeutics, 72,* 51-81.

Bates, C., Connolly, G. N., & Jarvis, M. (1999). *Tobacco additives: Cigarette engineering and nicotine addiction.* London: Imperial Cancer Research Fund, Action on Smoking and Health.

Bauer, U. E., Johnson, T. M., Hopkins, R. S., & Brooks, R. G. (2000). Changes in youth cigarette use and intention following implementation of a tobacco control program: Finding from the Florida Youth Tobacco Survey, 1998-2000. *Journal of the American Medical Association, 284,* 723-728.

Benowitz, N. L. (1993). Nicotine replacement therapy: What has been accomplished—Can we do better? *Drugs, 45,* 157-170.

Benowitz, N. L. (1996). Pharmacology of nicotine: Addiction and therapeutics. *Annual Review of Pharmacology and Toxicology, 36,* 597-613.

Benowitz, N. L. (1998a). Nicotine pharmacology and addiction. In N. L. Benowitz (Ed.), *Nicotine safety and toxicity* (pp. 3-16). New York: Oxford University Press.

Benowitz, N. L. (Ed.). (1998b). *Nicotine safety and toxicity.* New York: Oxford University Press.

Benowitz, N. L., & Henningfield, J. E. (1994). Establishing a nicotine threshold for addiction: The implications for tobacco regulation. *New England Journal of Medicine, 331,* 123-125.

Benowitz, N. L., Jacob, P., Kozlowski, L. T., & Yu, L. (1986). Impact of smoking fewer cigarettes on tar, nicotine, and carbon monoxide exposure. *New England Journal of Medicine, 315,* 1310-1313.

Benowitz, N. L., Porchet, H. P., Sheiner, L., & Jacob, P. (1988). Nicotine absorption and cardiovascular effects with smokeless tobacco use: Comparison with cigarettes and nicotine gum. *Clinical Pharmacology and Therapeutics, 44* (1), 23-28.

Biglan, A., Duncan, T. E., Ary, D. V., & Smolkowski, D. (1995). Peer and parental influences on adolescent tobacco use. *Journal of Behavioral Medicine, 18,* 315-330.

Bolinder, G. (1997). Smokeless tobacco: A less harmful alternative? In C. T. Bolliger & K. O. Fagerstrom (Eds.), *The tobacco epidemic* (pp. 199-212). Basel, Switzerland: Karger.

Bradford, J. A., Harlan, W. R., & Hanmer, H. R. (1936). Nature of cigarette smoke: Technique of experimental smoking. *Industrial and Engineering Chemistry, 28*(7), 836-839.

Brecher, E. M. (1972). *Licit and illicit drugs.* Mount Vernon, NY: Consumers Union.

Brecher, R., Brecher, E. M., & Editors of Consumers Report. (1963). *Consumers Union report on smoking and the public interest.* Mount Vernon, NY: Consumers Union.

Brigham, J. (1998). *Dying to quit: Why we smoke and how we stop.* Washington, DC: National Academy Press.

Brooks, J. E. (1953). *The mighty leaf: Tobacco through the centuries.* London: Alvin Redman.

Brown, D. (1999). Ashes to ashes: Richard Doll made the connection between smoking and cancer. *Washington Post,* p. C-1.

Bruntland, G. H. (2000). Achieving worldwide tobacco control. *Journal of the American Medical Association, 284,* 750-751.

Burns, D. M. (Ed.). (1998). *Cigars: Health effects and trends.* Bethesda, MD: National Cancer Institute.

Burns, D. M. (in press). *Population based smoking cessation: What works?* (NCI Monograph). Bethesda, MD: National Cancer Institute.

Burns, D. M., Benowitz, N. L., Connolly, G. N., Cummings, K. M., Davis, R. M., Henningfield, J. E., Shopland, D. R., & Warner, K. E. (1997). What should be the elements of any settlement with the tobacco industry? *Tobacco Control, 6,* 1-4.

Burns, D. M., Shanks, T., Major, J., & Thun, M. (in press). Evidence on disease risks in public health consequences of low yield cigarettes. In *Smoking and Tobacco Control Monograph, 13.* Washington, DC: National Cancer Institute.

Burns, D. M., Garfinkel, L., & Samet, J. M. (Eds.). (1997). *Changes in cigarette-related disease risks and their implication for prevention and control.* Bethesda, MD: National Cancer Institute.

Bynner, J. M. (1969). *The young smoker: A study of smoking among schoolboys carried out for the ministry of health* (Government Social Survey, SS383). London: Her Majesty's Stationery Office.

Byrd, G. D., Davis, R. A., Caldwell, W. S., Robinson, J. H., & deBethizy, J. D. (1997). A further study of FTC yield and nicotine absorption in smokers. *Psychopharmacology, 134,* 291-299.

Cahalan, D., & Room, R. (1974). *Problem drinking among American men.* (Rutgers Center of Alcohol Studies Monograph). New Brunswick, NJ: Rutgers Center of Alcohol Studies.

Callender, C. (1978). Fox. In B. G. Trigger (Ed.), *Handbook of North American Indians: Vol. 15. Northeast.* Washington, DC: Smithsonian Institution.

Centers for the Advancement of Health. (1998). *Treating tobacco dependence in the U.S.: Ad hoc group findings and recommendations.* Available: www.cfah.org.

Centers for Disease Control and Prevention. (1993). Mortality trends for selected smoking-related cancers and breast cancer—United States, 1950-1990. *Morbidity and Mortality Weekly Report, 42,* 857, 863-866.

Centers for Disease Control and Prevention. (1994). Reasons for tobacco use and symptoms of nicotine withdrawal among adolescent and young adult tobacco users—United States, 1993. *Morbidity and Mortality Weekly Report, 43,* 745-750.

Centers for Disease Control and Prevention. (1996a). Accessibility of tobacco products to youths aged 12-17 years—United States, 1989 and 1993. *Morbidity and Mortality Weekly Report, 45(6),* 125-130.

Centers for Disease Control and Prevention. (1996b). *CDC's Tobacco Use Prevention Program: Working toward a healthier future.* Washington, DC: U.S. Department of Health and Human Services.

Centers for Disease Control and Prevention. (1996c). Tobacco use and usual source of cigarettes among high school students—United States, 1995. *Morbidity and Mortality Weekly Report, 45(20),* 413-418.

Centers for Disease Control and Prevention. (1997). Cigar use among teenagers—United States, Massachusetts, and New York, 1996. *Morbidity and Mortality Weekly Report, 46(20),* 433-440.

Centers for Disease Control and Prevention. (1998a). State-specific prevalence among adults of current cigarette smoking and smokeless tobacco use and per capita tax-paid sales of cigarettes—United States, 1997. *Morbidity and Mortality Weekly Report, 47(43),* 922-926.

Centers for Disease Control and Prevention. (1998b). Tobacco use among high school students—United States, 1997. *Morbidity and Mortality Weekly Report, 47,* 229-233.

Centers for Disease Control and Prevention. (1998c). Youth behavior risk surveillance—United States, 1997. *Morbidity and Mortality Weekly Report, 47(SS-3),* 1-89.

Centers for Disease Control and Prevention. (2000a). *Current smokeless tobacco use among men aged 18 years and older—United States, 1992-1993.* Retrieved January 2, 2001, from the World Wide Web: www.cdc.gov/tobacco/research_data/spit/sltmen.htm

Centers for Disease Control and Prevention. (2000b). *Incidence of initiation of cigarette smoking among U.S. teens.* Retrieved January 2, 2001, from the World Wide Web: www.cdc.gov/tobacco/research_data/youth/initfact.htm

Centers for Disease Control and Prevention. (2000c). Tobacco use among middle and high school students—United States, 1999. *Morbidity and Mortality Weekly Report, 49(3),* 49-53.

Centers for Disease Control and Prevention. (2000d). Use of FDA-approved pharmacological treatments for tobacco dependence—United States, 1984-1988. *Morbidity and Mortality Weekly Report, 49*(29), 665-668.

Chapman, S. (1999). Where there's smoke there's fire. *Tobacco Control, 8,* 12-13.

Cohen, J. B. (1992). Research and policy issues in Ringold and Calfee's treatment of cigarette health claims. *Journal of Public Policy and Marketing, 11,* 82-86.

Cohen, S., Lichtenstein, E., Prochaska, J. O., Ross, J. S., Gritz, E. R., Carr, C. R., Orleans, C. T., Schoenbach, V. J., Biener, L., Abrams, D., DiClemente, C., Curry, S., Marlatt, G.A., Cummings, K. M., Emont, S. L., Giovino, G., & Ossip-Klein, D. (1989). Debunking myths about self-quitting: Evidence from 10 prospective studies of persons who attempt to quit smoking by themselves. *American Psychologist, 44,* 1355-1365.

Collishaw, N. E., & Lopez, A. D. (1996). *The tobacco epidemic: A global pubic health emergency.* Geneva: World Health Organization. Available: www.who.int/archives/tohalert/apr96/fulltext. html

Committee on Energy and Commerce, U.S. House of Representatives. (1988). *Health consequences of smoking: Nicotine addiction.* Hearings before the Subcommittee on Health and Environment of the Committee on Energy and Commerce, July 29, 1988. (Serial No. 100-169). Washington DC: Government Printing Office.

Committee on Energy and Commerce, U.S. House of Representatives. (1995). *Regulation of tobacco products (Part 1).* Hearings before the Subcommittee on Health and Environment of the Committee on Energy and Commerce, March 25 and April 14, 1994 (Serial No. 103-149). Washington, DC: Government Printing Office.

Conference on Tobacco Dependence: Innovative Regulatory Approaches to Reduce Death and Disease. (1998). *Food and Drug Law Journal, 53*(1; Special issue), 1-137.

Connolly, G. N. (1995). The marketing of nicotine addiction by one oral snuff manufacturer. *Tobacco Control, 4,* 73-79.

Corrigall, W. A. (1999). Nicotine self-administration in animals as a dependence model. *Nicotine & Tobacco Research, 1,* 11-20.

Corrigall, W. A., & Coen, K. M. (1989). Nicotine maintains robust self-administration in rats on a limited-access schedule. *Psychopharmacology, 99,* 473-478.

Corrigall, W. A., Franklin, K. B. J., Coen, K. M., & Clarke, P. B. S. (1992). The mesolimbic dopamine system is implicated in the reinforcing effects of nicotine. *Psychopharmacology, 107,* 285-289.

Cox, H. (2000). *The global cigarette: Origins and evolution of British American Tobacco, 1880-1945.* Guilford and King's Lynn, UK: Oxford University Press.

Cronk, C. E., & Sarvela, P. D. (1997). Alcohol, tobacco, and other drug use among rural/small town and urban youth: A secondary analysis of the Monitoring the Future data set. *American Journal of Public Health, 87,* 760-764.

Dale, L. C., Schroeder, D. R., Wolter, T. D., Croghan, I. T., Hurt, R. D., & Offord, K. P. (1998). Weight change after smoking cessation using variable doses of transdermal nicotine replacement. *Journal of General Internal Medicine, 13,* 9-15.

Dickson, S. A. (1954). *Panacea or precious bane: Tobacco in sixteenth-century literature.* New York: New York Public Library.

Doll, R., & Hill, A. B. (1950). Smoking and carcinoma of the lung: A preliminary report. *British Medical Journal, 2,* 739-748.

Doll, R., & Hill, A. B. (1954). The mortality of doctors in relation to their smoking habits: A preliminary report. *British Medical Journal, 1,* 1451-1455.

Douglas, C. (1998). Taking aim at the bull's-eye: The nicotine in tobacco products. *Tobacco Control, 7,* 215-218.

Elwa, C. (1974). *The book of pipes and tobacco.* New York: Random House.

Everett, S. A., Giovino, G. A., Warren, C. W., Crossett, L., & Kann, L. (1998). Other substance use among high school students who use tobacco. *Journal of Adolescent Health, 23,* 289-296.

Farkas, A. J., Distefan, J. M, Choi, W. S., Gilpin, E. A., & Pierce, J. P. (1999). Does parental smoking cessation discourage adolescent smoking? *Preventive Medicine, 28,* 213-218.

Farkas, A. J., Gilpin, E. A., White, M. M., & Pierce, J. P. (2000). Association between household and workplace smoking restrictions and adolescent smoking. *Journal of the American Medical Association, 284,* 717-722.

Federal Trade Commission. (1997). *Report to Congress: Pursuant to the Federal Cigarette Labelling and Advertising Act.* Washington, DC: Author.

Federal Trade Commission. (1999a). *1999 report on cigarette sales, advertising and promotion.* Washington, DC: Author.

Federal Trade Commission. (1999b). *Report to Congress: Cigar sales and advertising and promotional expenditures for calendar years 1996 and 1997.* Washington, DC: Author.

Ferrence, R. G., Slade, J., Room, R., & Pope, M. (Eds.). (2000). *Nicotine and public health.* Washington, DC: American Public Health Association.

Ferrence, R. G. (1990). *Deadly fashion: The rise and fall of cigarette smoking in North America* (Garland Studies in Historical Demography). New York: Garland.

Ferry, L. H., Grissino, L. M., & Runfola, P. S. (1999). Tobacco dependence curricula in US undergraduate medical education. *Journal of the American Medical Association, 282,* 825-829.

Feynman, R. (1988). *What do you care about what other people think? Further adventures of a curious character.* New York: Norton.

Fiore, M. C., Bailey, W. C., Cohen, S. J., et al. (1996). *Smoking cessation. Clinical practice guideline No. 18* (AHCPR Publication No. 96-0692). Rockville, MD: U.S. Department of Health and Human Services, Public Health Service, Agency for Health Care Policy and Research.

Fiore, M. C., Bailey W.C., & Cohen S .J., et al. (2000). *Treating tobacco use and dependence. Clinical practice guideline.* Rockville, MD: U.S. Department of Health and Human Services. Public Health Service.

Fischer, P. M., Schwartz, M. P., Richard, J. W., Jr., Goldstein, A. O., & Rojas, T. (1991). Brand logo recognition by children aged 3 to 6 years: Mickey Mouse and Old Joe the Camel. *Journal of the American Medical Association, 266,* 3145-3148.

Fix, A. J., Daughton, D., Kass, I., Smith, J. L., Wickiser, A., Golden, C. J., & Wass, A. R. (1983). Urinary alkalinization and smoking cessation. *Journal of Clinical Psychology, 39,* 617-623.

Food and Drug Administration. (1995). *Nicotine in cigarettes and smokeless tobacco products is a drug and these products are nicotine delivery devices under the Federal Food, Drug, and Cosmetic Act.* Appendices, Department of Health and Human Services, A1-A99. Available: www.access.gpo.gov/su_docs/fda/append.html

Food and Drug Administration. (1996). Regulations restricting the sale and distribution of cigarettes and smokeless tobacco to protect children and adolescents: Final Rule, CFR & 801, et al. *Federal Register, 61*(168), 44, 395-44, 445.

Garvey, A. J., Bliss, R. E., Hitchcock, J. L., Heinhold, J. W., & Rosner, B. (1992). Predictors of smoking relapse among self-quitters: A report from the Normative Aging Study. *Addictive Behaviors, 17,* 367.

Gerstein, D. R., & Levison, P. K. (1982). *Reduced tar and nicotine cigarettes: Smoking behavior and health* (Committee on Substance Abuse and Habitual Behavior, Commission on Behavioral and Social Sciences and Education, National Research Council). Washington, DC: National Academy Press.

Giovino, G. A., Henningfield, J. E., Tomar, S. L., Escobedo, L. G., & Slade, J. (1995). Epidemiology of tobacco use and dependence. *Epidemiologic Reviews, 17,* 48-65.

Giovino, G. A., Shelton, D. M., & Schooley, M. W. (1993). Trends in cigarette smoking cessation in the United States. *Tobacco Control, 2*(Suppl. 3), S3.

Giovino, G. A., Tomar, S. L., Reddy, M. N., Peddicord, J. P., Zhu, B. P., Escobedo, L. G., & Eriksen, M. P. (1996). Attitudes, knowledge, and beliefs about low-yield cigarettes among adolescents and adults. In *The FTC method for determining tar, nicotine, and carbon monoxide yields of US cigarettes: Report of the NCI Expert Committee* (pp. 39-57). Bethesda, MD: U.S. Department of Health & Human Services, National Cancer Institute.

Gladwell, M. (2000). *The tipping point.* New York: Little, Brown.

Glantz, S. A., Slade, J., Bero, L. A., Hanauer, P., & Barnes, D. E. (Eds.). (1996). *The cigarette papers.* Berkeley: University of California Press.

Gold, M. S. (1993). *Cocaine.* New York: Plenum Publishing.

Goldberg, S. R., Spealman, R. D., & Goldberg, D. M. (1981). Persistent behavior at high rates maintained by intravenous self-administration of nicotine. *Science, 24,* 573-575.

Goldstein, A. (1994). *Addiction: From biology to drug policy.* New York: Freeman.

Goodman, J. (1993). *Tobacco in history: The cultures of dependence.* London: Routledge.

Griffiths, R. R., Bigelow, G. E., & Henningfield, J. E. (1980). Similarities in animal and human drug-taking behavior. In N. K. Mello (Ed.), *Advances in substance abuse* (pp. 1-90). Greenwich, CT: JAI.

Grunberg, N. E. (1992). Cigarette smoking and body weight: A personal journey through a complex field. *Health Psychology, 11,* 26-31.

Grunberg, N. E., & Kozlowski, L. T. (1986). Alkaline therapy as an adjunct to smoking cessation programs. *International Journal of Biosocial Research, 8*(1), 43-52.

Hall, S. M., Tunstall, C. D., Vila, K. L., & Duffy, J. (1992). Weight gain prevention and smoking cessation: Cautionary findings. *American Journal of Public Health, 82,* 799-803.

Hammond, E. C., Garfinkel, L., Seidman, H., & Lew, E. A. (1976). Tar and nicotine content of cigarette smoke in relation to death rates. *Environmental Research, 12*(3), 263-274.

Hatsukami, D. K., & Severson, H. H. (1999). Oral spit tobacco: Addiction, prevention and treatment. *Nicotine & Tobacco Research, 1,* 21-44.

Hazan, A. R., & Glantz, S. A. (1995). Current trends in tobacco use on prime-time fictional television. *American Journal of Public Health, 85,* 116-117.

Hazan, A. R., Lipton, H. L., & Glantz, S. A. (1994). Popular films do not reflect current tobacco use. *American Journal of Public Health, 84,* 998-1000.

Heishman, S. J., Kozlowski, L. T., & Henningfield, J. E. (1997). Nicotine addiction: Implications for public policy. *Journal of Social Issues, 53,* 13-33.

Henningfield, J. E. (1992). Occasional drug use: Comparing nicotine with other addictive drugs. *Tobacco Control, 1,* 161-162.

Henningfield, J. E. (1997). Postscript. *Tobacco Control, 6*(Suppl.), S98-S99.

Henningfield, J. E. (2000). Tobacco dependence treatment: Scientific challenges; public health opportunities. *Tobacco Control, 9*(Suppl. I), I3-I10.

Henningfield, J. E., Benowitz, N. L., Slade, J., Houston, T. P., Davis, R. M., & Deitchman, S. D. (1998). Reducing the addictiveness of cigarettes. *Tobacco Control, 7,* 281-293.

Henningfield, J. E., Clayton, R., & Pollin, W. (1990). Involvement of tobacco in alcoholism and illicit drug use. *British Journal of Addiction, 85,* 279-292.

Henningfield, J. E., Cohen, C., & Slade, J. D. (1991). Is nicotine more addictive than cocaine? *British Journal of Addiction, 86,* 565-570.

Henningfield, J. E., Fant, R. V., Radzius, A., & Frost, S. (1999). Nicotine concentration, smoke pH and whole tobacco aqueous pH of some cigar brands and types popular in the United States. *Nicotine & Tobacco Research, 1,* 163-168.

Henningfield, J. E., Fant, R. V., Shiffman, S., & Gitchell, J. (2000). Tobacco dependence: Scientific and public health basis of treatment. *Economics of Neuroscience, 2*(2), 42-46.

Henningfield, J. E., Michaelides, T., & Sussman, S. (2000). Developing treatment for tobacco addicted youth: Issues and challenges. *Journal of Child and Adolescent Substance Abuse, 9,* 5-26.

Henningfield, J. E., Miyasato, K., & Jasinski, D. R. (1985). Abuse liability and pharmacodynamic characteristcis of intravenous and inhaled nicotine. *Journal of Pharmacology and Experimental Therapeutics, 234,* 1-12.

Henningfield, J. E., Schuh, L. M., & Heishman, S. J. (1995). Pharmacological determinants of cigarette smoking. In P. B. S. Clarke, M. Quik, F. X. Adlkofer, & K. Thurau (Eds.), *Effects of nicotine on biological systems II, International Symposium on nicotine* (pp. 247-256). Basel, Switzerland: Birkhauser Verlag.

Henningfield, J. E., Schuh, L. M., & Jarvik, M. E. (1995). Pathophysiology of tobaccco dependence. In F. E. Bloom, & D. J. Kupfer (Eds.), *Psychopharmacology: The fourth generation of progress* (pp. 1715-1729). New York: Raven.

Henningfield, J. E., & Slade, J. (1998). Tobacco dependence medications: Public health and regulatory issues. *Food and Drug Law Journal, 53*(Suppl.), 75-114.

Henningfield, J. E., Stapleton, J. M., Benowitz, N. L., & London, E. D. (1993). Higher levels of nicotine in arterial than in venous blood after cigarette smoking. *Drug and Alcohol Dependence, 33,* 23-29.

Herling, S., & Kozlowski, L. T. (1988). The importance of direct questions about inhalation and daily intake in the evaluation of pipe and cigar smokers. *Preventive Medicine, 17,* 73-78.

Herndon, M. (1957). *Tobacco in colonial Virginia.* Williamsburg: Virginia 350th Anniversary Celebration Corporation.

Hills, L. R. (1993). *How to do things right: The memoirs of a fussy man.* Boston: Godine.

Hilts, P. J. (1998). *Smoke screen.* New York: Diane Publishing.

Hirschhorn, N. (2000). Shameful science: Four decades of the German tobacco industry's hidden research on smoking and health. *Tobacco Control, 9,* 242-247.

Hoffman, D., & Hoffman, I. (1997). The changing cigarette, 1950-1995. *Journal of Toxicology and Environmental Health, 50,* 307-364.

Hughes, J. R. (in press). Impact of medications on smoking cessation. In D. Burns (Ed.), *Population impact of smoking cessation interventions* (NCI Monograph). Bethesda, MD: National Cancer Institute.

Hughes, J. R., Goldstein, M. G., Hurt, R. D., & Shiffman, S. (1999). Recent advances in the pharmacotherapy of smoking. *Journal of the American Medical Association, 281,* 72-76.

Hughes, J. R., & Hatsukami, D. (1986). Signs and symptoms of tobacco withdrawal. *Archives of General Psychiatry, 43,* 289-294.

Hughes, J. R., Higgins, S. T., & Bickel, W. K. (1994). Nicotine withdrawal versus other drug withdrawal symptoms: Similarities and dissimilarities. *Addiction, 89,* 1461-1470.

Hurt, R. D., & Robertson, C. R. (1998). Prying open the door to the tobacco industry's secrets about nicotine. *Journal of the American Medical Association, 280* (13) 1173-1181.

Institute of Medicine. (1997). *Dispelling the myths about drug addiction.* Washington, DC: National Academy Press.

Jackson, C., Henriksen, L., Dickinson, D., & Levine, D. W. (1997). The early use of alcohol and tobacco: Its relation to children's competence and parents' behavior. *American Journal of Public Health, 87,* 359-364.

Jaffe, J. H. (1990). Tobacco smoking and nicotine dependence. In S. Wonnacott, M. A. H. Russell, & I. P. Stolerman (Eds.), *Nicotine psychopharmacology: Molecular, cellular, and behavioural aspects* (pp. 1-37). Oxford, UK: Oxford University Press.

James, J. E. (1997). *Understanding caffeine: A biobehavioral analysis.* Thousand Oaks, CA: Sage.

Jarvik, M. E. (1995). Commentary. *Psychopharmacology,* 17, 18-20.

Jenkins, R. A., Quincy, R. B., & Guerin, M. R. (1979). Selected constituents in the smokes of U.S. commercial cigarettes: Tar, nicotine, carbon monoxide and carbon dioxide (Department of Energy Rep. No. ORNL/TM-6870).: Oak Ridge National Laboratory (NTIS No. 22161). (Available from National Technical Information Service, Springfield, VA 22161.)

Joeres, R., Klinker, H., Heusler, H., Epping, J., Zilly, W., & Richter, E. (1988). Influence of smoking on caffeine elimination in healthy volunteers and in patients with alcoholic liver cirrhosis. *Hepatology, 8,* 575-579.

Johnston, B. D. (1977). The race, class, irreversibility hypotheses: Myths and research about heroin. In J. D. Rittenhouse (Ed.), *The epidemiology of heroin and other narcotics* (National Institute on Drug Abuse Research Monograph Series 16, pp. 51-60). Bethesda, MD: National Institute on Drug Abuse.

Kalant, H., Clarke, P., Corrigall, W., Ferrence, R. G., & Kozlowski, L. T. (1989). *Tobacco, nicotine, and addiction: A committee report prepared at the request of the Royal Society of Canada.* Ottawa, Ontario: Royal Society of Canada.

Kandel, D. B. (1980). Developmental stages in adolescent drug involvement. In D. J. Lettieri, M. Sayers, & H. W. Pearson (Eds.), *Theories of drug abuse: Selected contemporary perspectives* (NIDA Research Monograph No. 30; DHHS Publication No. ADM 80-967). Washington, DC: Government Printing Office.

Kandel, D. B., & Yamaguchi, K. (1985). Developmental patterns of the use of legal, illegal, and medically prescribed psychotropic drugs from adolescence to young adulthood. In C. L. Jones & R. J. Battjes (Eds.), *Etiology of drug abuse: Implications for prevention* (NIDA Research Monograph No. 56; DHHS Publication No. ADM 85-1335). Washington, DC: Government Printing Office.

Katims, D. S., & Zapata, J. T. (1993). Gender differences in substance use among Mexican-American school-age children. *Journal of School Health, 63,* 397-401.

Kendler, K. S., Neale, M. C., Sullivan, P., Corey, L. A., Gardner, C. O., & Prescott, C. A. (1999). A population-based twin study in women of smoking initiation and nicotine dependence. *Psychological Medicine, 29,* 299-308.

Kessler, D. A. (1999). Where there's smoke. *Talk,* 183-229.

Kessler, D. (2001). *A question of intent: The great American battle with a deadly industry.* New York, NY: PublicAffairs.

Kessler, D. A. (2000, April 3). Time to act on cigarettes. *Washington Post,* p. A17.

Kessler, D. A., Zeller, M. R., Natanblut, J. P., Lorraine, C. C., Thompson, L. J., & Schults, W. B. (1996). The Food and Drug Administration's regulation of tobacco products. *New England Journal of Medicine, 335*(13) 988-994.

King, C., Siegal, M., Celebucki, C., & Connolly, G. N. (1998). Adolescent exposure to cigarette advertising in magazines. *Journal of the American Medical Association, 279,* 516-520.

King James I. (1954). *The counter-blaste against tobacco.* London: Rodale. (Original work published in 1604).

Kluger, R. (1996). *Ashes to ashes: America's hundred-year cigarette war, the public health, and the unabashed triumph of Philip Morris.* New York: Knopf.

Koop, C. E. (1998, March 8). Don't forget the smokers. *Washington Post,* p. C7.

Koopmans, J. R., van Doornen, L. J., & Boomsma, D. I. (1997). Association between alcohol use and smoking in adolescent and young adult twins: A bivariate genetic analysis. *Alcohol: Clinical and Experimental Research, 21,* 537-546.

Kozlowski, L. T. (1976). Effects of caffeine consumption on nicotine consumption. *Psychopharmacology, 47,* 165-168.

Kozlowski, L. T. (1981). Tar and nicotine delivery of cigarettes: What a difference a puff makes. *Journal of the American Medical Association, 245*(2), 158-159.

Kozlowski, L. T. (1982). The determinants of tobacco use: Cigarettes in the context of other forms of tobacco use. *Canadian Journal of Public Health, 73,* 236-241.

Kozlowski, L. T. (1986). Pack size, self-reported smoking rates and public health. *American Journal of Public Health, 76,* 1337-1338.

Kozlowski, L. T. (1987). Finding help to quit cigarettes. *Harvard Medical School Health Letter, 13,* 6-7.

Kozlowski, L. T. (1989). Evidence for limits on the acceptability of lowest tar cigarettes. *American Journal of Public Health, 79,* 198-199.

Kozlowski, L. T. (1991). Rehabilitating a genetic perspective in the study of tobacco and alcohol use. *British Journal of Addiction, 86,* 517-520.

Kozlowski, L. T. (2000). Some lessons from the history of American tobacco advertising and its regulation in the 20th century. In R. Ferrence, J. Slade, R. Room, & M. Pope (Eds.), *Nicotine and public health.* Washington, DC: American Public Health Association.

Kozlowski, L. T., Appel, C-P., Frecker, R. C., & Khouw, V. (1982). Nicotine, a prescribable drug available without prescription. *Lancet, 1,* 334.

Kozlowski, L. T., Coambs, R. C., Ferrence, R. G., & Adlaf, E. (1989). Preventing smoking and other drug use: Let the buyer beware and the interventions be apt. *Canadian Journal of Public Health, 80*(6), 452-456.

Kozlowski, L. T., & Ferrence, R. G. (1990). Statistical control in research on alcohol and tobacco: An example from research on alcohol and mortality. *British Journal of Addiction, 85,* 271-278.

Kozlowski, L. T., Frecker, R. C., Khouw, V., & Pope, M. (1980). The misuse of "less-hazardous" cigarettes and its detection: Hole-blocking of ventilated filters. *American Journal of Public Health, 70,* 1202-1203.

Kozlowski, L. T., Goldberg, M. E., Sweeney, C. T., Palmer, R. F., Pillitteri, J. L., White, E. L., & Stine, M. M. (1999). Smoker reactions to a "radio message" that light cigarettes are as dangerous as regulars. *Nicotine & Tobacco Research, 1,* 67-76.

Kozlowski, L. T., Goldberg, M. E., Yost, B. A., Ahern, F. M., Aronson, K. R., & Sweeney, C. T. (1997). Smokers are unaware of the filter vents now on most cigarettes: Results of a national survey. *Tobacco Control, 6,* 1-6.

Kozlowski, L. T., Goldberg, M. E., Yost, B. A., White, E. L., Sweeney, C. S., & Pillitteri, J. L. (1998). Smokers' misperceptions of light and ultra-light cigarettes may keep them smoking. *American Journal of Preventive Medicine, 15*(1), 9-16.

Kozlowski, L. T., & Harford, M. A. (1976). On the significance of never using a drug: An example from cigarette smoking. *Journal of Abnormal Psychology, 85*(4), 433-434.

Kozlowski, L. T., Heatherton, T. F., Frecker, R. C., & Nolte, H. E. (1989). Self-selected blocking of vents on low-yield cigarettes. *Pharmacology, Biochemistry and Behavior, 33,* 815-819.

Kozlowski, L. T., Henningfield, J. E., Keenan, R. M., Lei, H., Leigh, G., Jelinek, L., Pope, M. A., & Haertzen, C. A. (1993). Patterns of alcohol, cigarette, and caffeine and other drug use in two drug abusing populations. *Journal of Substance Abuse Treatment, 10,* 171-179.

Kozlowski, L. T., & Herman, C. P. (1984). The interaction of psychosocial and biological determinants of tobacco use: More on the boundary model. *Journal of Applied Social Psychology, 14,* 244-256.

Kozlowski, L. T., Jelinek, L., & Pope, M. A. (1986). Cigarette smoking among alcoholics: A continuing and neglected problem. *Canadian Journal of Public Health, 77,* 205-207.

Kozlowski, L. T., Mehta, N. Y., Sweeney, C. T., Richter, P., & Giovino, G. (1997). Filter ventilation levels in selected U.S. cigarettes—1997. *Morbidity and Mortality Weekly Report, 46*(44), 1043-1047.

Kozlowski, L. T., Mehta, N. Y., Sweeney, C. T., Schwartz, S. S., Vogler, G. P., Jarvis, M. J., & West, R. J. (1998). Filter ventilation and nicotine content of tobacco in cigarettes from Canada, the United Kingdom, and the United States. *Tobacco Control, 7,* 369-375.

Kozlowski, L. T., & O'Connor, R. J. (in press). Official cigarette tar tests are misleading: Use a two-stage, compensating test. *Lancet, 355,* 2159-2161.

Kozlowski, L. T., O'Connor, R. J., & Sweeney, C. T. (2000). Cigarette design. In *Smoking and Tobacco Control Monograph, 13.* Washington, DC: National Cancer Institute.

Kozlowski, L. T., Porter, C. Q., Orleans, C. T., Pope, M. A., & Heatherton, T. (1994). Predicting smoking cessation with self-reported measures of nicotine dependence: FTQ, FTND, and HSI. *Drug and Alcohol Dependence, 34,* 211-216.

Kozlowski, L. T., Rickert, W. S., Pope, M. A., Robinson, J. C., & Frecker, R. C. (1982). Estimating the yield to smokers of tar, nicotine, and carbon monoxide from the "lowest yield" ventilated-filter cigarettes. *British Journal of Addiction, 77,* 159-165.

Kozlowski, L. T., Rickert, W., Robinson, J., & Grunberg, N. E. (1980). Have tar and nicotine yields of cigarettes changed? *Science, 209,* 1550-1551.

Kozlowski, L. T., Skinner, W., Kent, C., & Pope, M. A. (1989). Prospects for smoking treatment in individuals seeking treatment for alcohol and other drug problems. *Addictive Behaviors, 14,* 273-278.

Kozlowski, L. T., White, E. L., Sweeney, C. T., Yost, B. A., Ahern, F. M., & Goldberg, M. E. (1998). Few smokers know their cigarettes have filter vents. *American Journal of Public Health, 88*(4), 681-682.

Kozlowski, L. T., & Wilkinson, D. A. (1987). Use and misuse of the concept of craving by alcohol, tobacco, and drug researchers. *British Journal of Addiction, 82,* 31-45.

Kozlowski, L. T., Wilkinson, D. A., Skinner, W., Kent, C., Franklin, T., & Pope, M. (1989). Comparing tobacco cigarette dependence with other drug dependencies: Greater or equal "difficulty quitting" and "urges to use," but less "pleasure" from cigarettes. *Journal of the American Medical Association, 261*(6), 896-901.

Kozlowski, L. T., Yost, B., Stine, M. M., & Celebucki, C. (2000). Massachusetts' advertising against light cigarettes appears to change beliefs and behavior. *American Journal of Preventive Medicine, 18*(4), 339-342.

Kreek, M. J. (1987). Multiple drug abuse patterns and medical consequences. In H. Y. Meltzer (Ed.), *Psychopharmacology: The third generation of progress.* New York: Raven.

Kreek, M. J. (1992). Rationale for maintenance pharmacotherapy of opiate dependence. In C. P. O'Brien & J. H. Jaffe (Eds.), *Addictive States.* New York: Raven.

La Barre, W. (1972). *The ghost dance: Origins of religion.* New York: Dell.

Langley, J. N. (1906). On nerve endings and special excitable substances in cells (A Croonian Lecture). *Proceedings of the Royal Society of London, 78,* 170-194.

Lefkowitz, R. J., Hoffman, B. B., & Taylor, P. (1996). Neurotransmission: The autonomic and somatic motor nervous systems. In P. B. Molinoff, & R. W. Ruddon (Eds.), *Goodman and Gilman's the pharmacological basis of therapeutics* (9th ed., pp. 105-139). New York: McGraw-Hill.

Leventhal, H., Glynn, K., & Fleming, R. (1987). Is the smoking decision an "informed choice"? Effect of smoking risk factors on smoking beliefs. *Journal of the American Medical Association, 257,* 3373-3376.

Lévi-Strauss, C. (1973). *From honey to ashes. Introduction to a science of mythology: 2.* New York: Harper & Row.

Lewine, H. (1970). *Good-bye to all that.* New York: McGraw-Hill.

Lloyd, B., & Lucas, K. (1998). *Smoking in adolescence: Images and identities.* New York: Routledge.

Lynch, B. S., & Bonnie, R. J. (Eds.). (1994). *Growing up tobacco free: Preventing nicotine addiction in children and youths.* Washington, DC: Institute of Medicine, National Academy Press.

Mackay, J., & Crofton, J. (1996). Tobacco and the developing world. *British Medical Bulletin, 52,* 206-221.

McNeill, A. D., Jarvis, M. J., Stapleton, J. A., West, R. J., & Bryant, A. (1989). Nicotine intake in young smokers: Longitudinal study of saliva cotinine concentrations. *American Journal of Public Health, 79,* 172-175.

McNeill, A. D., West, R. J., Jarvis, M. J., Jackson, P., & Bryant, A. (1986). Cigarette withdrawal symptoms in adolescent smokers. *Psychopharmacology, 90,* 533-536.

Miller, W., & Rollnick, S. (1991). *Motivational interviewing: Preparing people to change addictive behavior.* New York: Guilford.

Moore, D. W. (1999, October 14). Americans agree with Philip Morris: Smoking is harmful (Poll Releases). *Gallup News Services.*

Murray, J. A. H., Bradley, H., Craigie, W. A., & Onions, C. T. (Eds.). (1933). *New English dictionary on historical principles (Oxford English Dictionary).* Oxford, UK: Clarendon.

National Cancer Institute. (1997). *Changes in cigarette-related disease risks and their implication for prevention and control.* D. M. Burns, L. Garfinkel, & J. M. Samet (Eds.). Bethesda, MD: National Cancer Institute.

National Cancer Institute. (1998). *Cigars: Health effects and trends.* D. M. Burns (Ed.). Bethesda, MD: National Cancer Institute.

National Cancer Institute. (1999). *Health effects of exposure to environmental tobacco smoke.* Bethesda, MD: Author.

National Cancer Institute. (2000). *State and local legislative action to reduce tobacco use* (Smoking and Tobacco Control Monograph No. 11; NIH Publication No. 00-4804). Bethesda, MD: U.S. Department of Health and Human Services, National Institutes of Health, National Cancer Institute.

National Institute on Drug Abuse. (1991). National Household Survey on Drug Abuse: Main findings, 1990 (DHHS Publication ADM 91-1788). Rockville, MD: U.S. Department of Health and Human Services, Public Health Service; Alcohol, Drug Abuse, and Mental Health Administration.

Nothwehr, F., Lando, H. A., & Bobo, J. K. (1995). Alcohol and tobacco use in the Minnesota Heart Health Program. *Addictive Behaviors, 20,* 463-470.

Office of Smoking and Health. Retrieved from CDC website http://www.cdc.gov/tobacco/research_data/health_consequences/mortali.htm

Oh, H., Yamazaki, Y., & Kawata, C. (1998). Prevalence and a drug use development model for the study of adolescent drug use in Japan [English abstract, translated from Japanese]. *Nippon Koshu Eisei Zasshi, 45,* 870-882.

Ortiz, F. (1947). *Cuban counterpoint.* New York: Knopf.

Page, J. A. (1998). Federal regulation of tobacco products and products that treat tobacco dependence: Are the playing fields level? *Food and Drug Law Journal, 53*(Suppl.), 11-43.

Pangritz, O. (1984, July). Smoke elasticity, Session III. *Proceedings of the Smoking Behaviour-Marketing Conference* (p. 58). Montreal, Quebec, BAT Co. Retrieved January 2, 2001, from the World Wide Web: www.tobaccopapers.org/Conferences/84-Smoking-Behaviour-Marketing/84SBM-III-Elasticity.pdf

Parra-Medina, D. M., Talavera, G., Elder, J. P., & Woodruff, S. I. (1995). Role of cigarette smoking as a gateway drug to alcohol use in Hispanic junior high school students. *Journal of the National Cancer Institute Monographs, 18,* 83-86.

Parrott, S., Godfrey, C., Raw, M., West, R., & McNeill, A. (1998). Guidance for commissioners on the cost effectiveness of smoking cessation interventions. *Thorax, 53*(Suppl. 5, Pt. 2), S1-S38.

Participants of the Fourth Scarborough Conference on Preventive Medicine. (1985). Is there a future for lower-tar-yield cigarettes? *Lancet, 2,* 1111-1114.

Partington, W. (1925). *Smoke rings and roundelays: Blendings from prose and verse since Raleigh's time.* New York: Dodd, Mead.

Patterson, J. T. (1989). *The dread disease: Cancer and modern American culture.* Cambridge, MA: Harvard University Press.

Peeler, C. L. (1996). Cigarette testing and the Federal Trade Commission: A historical overview. In *The FTC method for determining tar, nicotine, and carbon monoxide yields of US cigarettes: Report of the NCI Expert Committee* (pp. 1-8). Bethesda, MD: U.S. Department of Health & Human Services, National Cancer Institute.

Pena, P., & l'Obel, M. (1571). *Stirpium adversaria nova* (Original in Library of Congress). Image produced by Bell & Howell Information and Learning Company as part of Early English Books Online. Inquiries may be made to: Bell & Howell Information and Learning Company, 300 North Zeeb Road, Ann Arbor, MI 48106-1346 USA. Telephone 734-761-7400; E-mail: info@bellhowell.infolearning.com; Web page: www.bellhowell.infolearning.com

Perkins, K. A., Donny, E., & Caggiula, A. R. (1999). Sex differences in nicotine effects and self-administration: Review of human and animal evidence. *Nicotine & Tobacco Research, 1,* 301-315.

Perkins, K. A., Sexton, J. E., DiMarco, A., Grobe, J. E., Scierka, A., & Stiller, R. L. (1995). Subjective and cardiovascular responses to nicotine combined with alcohol in male and female smokers. *Psychopharmacology, 119,* 205-212.

Phil, R. O., & Spiers, P. (1978). Individual characteristics in the etiology of drug abuse. In B. A. Maher (Ed.), *Progress in experimental psychopathology research* (Vol. 8, pp. 93-195). New York: Academic Press.

Piasecki, M., & Newhouse, P. A. (Eds.). (2000). *Nicotine in psychiatry: Psychopathology and emerging therapeutics.* Washington, DC: American Psychiatric Press.

Pierce, J. P., Choi, W. S., Gilpin, E. A., Farkas, A. J., & Berry, C. C. (1998). Tobacco industry promotion of cigarettes and adolescent smoking. *Journal of the American Medical Association, 279,* 511-515.

Pierce, J. P., Farkas, A. J., Evans, C., Berry, C. C., Choi, W. S., Roshrook, B., Johnson, M., & Bai, D. G. (1993). *Tobacco use in California 1992. A focus on preventing uptake in adolescents.* Sacramento, CA: Department of Health Services.

Pierce, J. P., Fiore, M. C., Novotny, T. E., Hatziandreu, E. J., & Davis, R. M. (1989). Trends in cigarette smoking in the United States, projections to the year 2000. *Journal of the American Medical Association, 261,* 61-65.

Pillitteri, J. L., Kozlowski, L. T., Sweeney, C. T., & Heatherton, T. (1997). Individual differences in the subjective effects of the first cigarette of the day: A self-report method of studying tolerance. *Experimental and Clinical Psychopharmacology, 5*(1), 83-90.

Pomerleau, O. F. (1995). Individual differences in sensitivity to nicotine: Implications for genetic research on nicotine dependence. *Behavior Genetics, 25,* 161-177.

Pomerleau, O. F., Collins, A. C., Shiffman, S., & Pomerleau, C. S. (1993). Why some people smoke and others do not: New perspectives. *Journal of Consulting and Clinical Psychology, 61,* 723-731.

Powley, T. L. (1977). The ventrometrial hypothalamic syndrome, satiety, and a cephalic phase hypothesis. *Psychological Review, 84,* 89-126.

Raw, M. (2000). *Kick the habit: How to stop smoking and stay stopped.* London: BBC Worldwide.

Raw, M., McNeill, A., & West, R. (1998). Smoking cessation guidelines for health professionals: A guide to effective smoking cessation interventions for the health care system. *Thorax, 53*(Suppl. 5, Pt. 1), S1-S19.

Richmond, R. L., Debono, D. S., Larcos, D., & Kehoe, L. (1998). Worldwide survey of education on tobacco in medical schools. *Tobacco Control, 7*(3), 247-252.

Rickert, W. S., Robinson, J. C., & Lawless, E. (1989). Limitations to potential uses for data based on the machine smoking of cigarettes: Cigarette smoke contents. In N. Wald, & P. Froggatt (Eds.), *Nicotine, smoking, and the low tar programme* (pp. 85-99). New York: Oxford University Press.

Rigotti, N. A., Lee, J. E., & Wechsler, H. (2000). US college students use of tobacco products. *Journal of the American Medical Association, 284,* 699-705.

Robert, J. C. (1949). *The story of tobacco in America.* Chapel Hill: University of North Carolina Press.

Robins, L. N. (1975). *A follow-up of Vietnam drug users.* Washington, DC: Special Action Office for Drug Abuse Prevention.

Robins, L. N. (1993). Vietnam veterans rapid recovery from heroin addiction: A fluke or normal expectation. *Addiction, 8,* 1041-1054.

Rogers, E. M. (1983). *Diffusion of innovations* (3rd ed.). New York: Free Press.

Royal College of Physicians. (2000). *Nicotine addiction in Britain: A report of the tobacco advisory group of the Royal College of Physicians.* London: Author.

Russell, M. A. H. (1971). Cigarette smoking: Natural history of a dependence disorder. *British Journal of Medical Psychology, 44,* 1-16.

Russell, M. A. H. (1990). The nicotine addiction trap: A 40-year sentence for four cigarettes. *British Journal of Addiction, 85,* 293-300.

Russell, M. A. H., & Feyerabend, C. (1978). Cigarette smoking: A dependence on high-nicotine boli. *Drug Metabolism Reviews, 8*(1), 29-57.

Schachter, S., Silverstein, B., Kozlowski, L. T., Perlick, D., Herman, C. P., & Liebling, B. (1977). Studies of the interaction of psychological and pharmacological determinants of smoking. *Journal of Experimental Psychology: General, 106*(1), 3-40.

Scherer, G. (1999). Smoking behaviour and compensation: A review of the literature. *Psychopharmacology 145,* 1-20.

Schneider, N. G., Lunell, E., Olmstead, R. E., & Fagerstrom, K. O. (1996). Clinical pharmacology of nasal nicotine delivery: A review and comparison to other nicotine systems. *Clinical Pharmacokinetics, 31,* 65-80.

Schoenborn, K. J., & Benson, V. (1988). *Relationships between smoking and other unhealthy habits: United States, 1985.* Washington, DC: Government Printing Office.

Schwartz, J. (1999, January 21). Reengineering the cigarette. *Washington Post Magazine,* pp. 9-24.

Shiffman, S., Gitchell, J., Pinney, J. M., Burton, S. L., Kemper, K. E., & Lara, E. A. (1997). Public health benefit of over-the-counter nicotine medications. *Tobacco Control, 6,* 306-310.

Shoaib, M., Swanner, L. S., Yasar, S., & Goldberg, S. R. (1999). Chronic caffeine exposure potentiates nicotine self-administration in rats. *Psychopharmacology, 142,* 327-333.

Silverstein, B., Feld, S., & Kozlowski, L. T. (1980). The availability of low-tar cigarettes as a cause of cigarette smoking among teenage females. *Journal of Health and Social Behavior, 21,* 383-388.

Silverstein, B., Kelly, E., Swan, J., & Kozlowski, L. T. (1982). Physiological predisposition towards becoming a cigarette smoker: Experimental evidence for a sex difference. *Addictive Behaviors, 7,* 83-86.

Sinclair, H. K., Bond, C. M., Lennox, A. S., Silcock, J., Winfield, A. J., & Donnan, P. T. (1998). Training pharmacists and pharmacy assistants in the stage-of-change model of smoking cessation: A randomized controlled trial in Scotland. *Tobacco Control, 7*(3), 253-262.

Slade, J. (1993). Nicotine delivery devices. In C. T. Orleans & J. Slade (Eds.), *Nicotine addiction: Principles and management* (pp. 3-23). New York: Oxford University Press.

Slade, J., Bero, L. A., Hanauer, P., Barnes, D. E., & Glantz, S. A. (1995). Nicotine and addiction: The Brown and Williamson documents. *Journal of the American Medical Association 274*(3), 225-233.

Slade, J., & Henningfield, J. E. (1998). Tobacco product regulation: Context and issues. *Food and Drug Law Journal, 53*(Suppl.), 43-74.

Smart, R. G., & Adlaf, E. M. (1987). *Alcohol and other drug use among Ontario students.* Toronto: Addiction Research Foundation.

Smoking kills: A white paper on tobacco. (1998). Presented to Parliament by the Secretary of State for Health and the Secretaries of State for Scotland, Wales and Northern Ireland. London: Her Majesty's Stationery Office: Available: http://www.official-documents.co.uk

Snell, W. (1999). *Structural changes in U.S. tobacco farms.* Retrieved December 11, 2000, from the World Wide Web: www.uky.edu/Agriculture/TobaccoEcon/publications/structural.pdf

Stallings, M. C., Hewitt, J. K., Beresford, T., Health, A. C., & Eaves, L. J. (1999). A twin study of drinking and smoking onset and latencies from first use to regular use. *Behavioral Genetics, 29,* 409-421.

Stolerman, I. P. (1999). Interspecies consistency in the behavioral pharmacology of nicotine dependence. *Behavioral Pharmacology, 10,* 559-580.

Strain, E. C., Mumford, G. K., Silverman, K., & Griffiths, R. R. (1994). Caffeine dependence syndrome. Evidence from case histories and experimental evaluations. *Journal of the American Medical Association, 272,* 1043-1048.

Substance Abuse and Mental Health Services Administration. (1999). *National Household Survey on Drug Abuse Series: H-10. National Household Survey on Drug Abuse: Population Estimates, 1998* (DHHS Pub. No. SMA 99-3327). Washington, DC: Government Printing Office.

Sussman, S., Dent, C. W., Mestel-Rauch, J., Johnson, C. A., Hansen, W., & Flay, B. R. (1988). Adolescent nonsmokers, triers, and regular smokers' estimates of cigarette smoking prevalence: When do overestimates occur and by whom? *Journal of Applied Social Psychology, 18*(7), 537-551.

Sutherland, I., & Willner, P. (1998). Patterns of alcohol, cigarette and illicit drug use in English adolescents. *Addiction, 93,* 1199-1208.

Swan, G. E., Carmelli, D., & Cardon, L. R. (1996). The consumption of tobacco, alcohol, and coffee in caucasian male twins: A multivariate genetic analysis. *Journal of Substance Abuse, 8,* 19-31.

Swan, G. E., Carmelli, D., & Cardon, L. R. (1997). Heavy consumption of cigarettes, alcohol and coffee in male twins. *Journal of Studies on Alcohol, 58,* 182-190.

Sweanor, D. (2000). Regulatory imbalance between medicinal and non-medicinal nicotine. *Addiction, 95*(1), S25-S28.

Swedberg, M. B. D., Henningfield, J. E., & Goldberg, S. R. (1990). Nicotine dependency: Animal studies. In S. Wonnacott, M. A. H. Russell, & I. P. Stolerman (Eds.), *Nicotine psychopharmacology: Molecular, cellular and behavioral aspects* (pp. 38-76). Oxford, UK: Oxford University Press.

Sweeney, C. T., Kozlowski, L. T., & Parsa, P. (1999). Effect of filter vent blocking on carbon monoxide exposure from selected lower tar cigarette brands. *Pharmacology, Biochemistry and Behavior, 63*(1), 167-173.

Thomas, B. S. (1996). A path analysis of gender differences in adolescent onset of alcohol, tobacco and other drug use (ATOD), reported ATOD use and adverse consequences of ATOD use. *Journal of Addictive Diseases, 15,* 33-52.

Thun, M. J., Day-Lally, C. A., Calle, E. E., Flanders, W. D., & Heath, C. W. (1995). Excess mortality among cigarette smokers: Changes in a 20-year interval. *American Journal of Public Health, 85,* 1223-1230.

Tomasello, T. (1997). Two pharmacy-practice models for implementing the AHCPR smoking cessation guideline. *Tobacco Control, 6*(Suppl.), S36-S38.

Tooker, E. (Ed.). (1979). *Native North American spirituality of the Eastern woodlands.* London: SPCK.

Top ten advertising icons of the century. (1999). *Advertising Age.* Retrieved December 11, 2000, from the World Wide Web: www.adage.com/century/icon01.html

Tyas, S. L., & Pederson, L. L. (1998). Psychosocial factors related to adolescent smoking: A critical review of the literature. *Tobacco Control, 7*(4), 409-433.

United Kingdom, House of Commons, Health Committee. (2000). *Second report: The tobacco industry and the health risks of Smoking.* London: Stationery Office Limited.

U.S. Department of Health, Education, and Welfare. (1964). *Smoking and health: Report of the Advisory Committee to the surgeon general of the Public Health Service.* Washington, DC: Author..

U.S. Department of Health, Education, and Welfare. (1979). *Smoking and health: A report of the surgeon general* (DHEW Publication No. PHS 79-50066). Washington, DC: U.S. Department of Health, Education, and Welfare, Public Health Service, Office of the Assistant Secretary for Health, Office on Smoking and Health.

U.S. Department of Health and Human Services. (1980). *The health consequences of smoking for women: A report of the surgeon general.* Washington, DC: U.S. Department of Health and Human Services, Public Health Service, Office of the Assistant Secretary for Health, Office on Smoking and Health.

U.S. Department of Health and Human Services. (1983). *Why people smoke cigarettes* (PHS Publication No. 83-50915). Rockville, MD: Author.

U.S. Department of Health and Human Services. (1986). *The health consequences of using smokeless tobacco: A report of the Advisory Committee to the surgeon general.* Washington, DC: Author.

U.S. Department of Health and Human Services. (1988). *Nicotine addiction—A report of the surgeon general.* Washington, DC: Author.

U.S. Department of Health and Human Services. (1989). *Reducing the health consequences of smoking: 25 years of progress—A report of the surgeon general.* Washington, DC: Author.

U.S. Department of Health and Human Services. (1990). *The health benefits of smoking cessation—A report of the surgeon general.* Washington, DC: Author.

U.S. Department of Health and Human Services. (1994). *Preventing tobacco use among young people—A report of the surgeon general.* Washington, DC: Author.

von Gernet, A. (2000). Origins of nicotine use and the global diffusion of tobacco. In R. Ferrence, J. Slade, R. Room, & M. Pope (Eds.), *Nicotine and public health.* Washington, DC: American Public Health Association.

Wakefield, M. A., Chaloupka, F. J., Kaufman, N. J., Orleans, C. T., Barker, D. C., & Ruel, E. E. (2000). Effect of restrictions on smoking at home, at school, and in public places on teenage smoking: Cross-sectional study. *British Medical Journal, 321,* 333-337.

Wald, N. J., & Watt, H. C. (1997). Prospective study of effect of switching from cigarettes to pipes or cigars on mortality from three smoking-related diseases. *British Medical Journal, 314,* 1860-1863.

Warner, K. E., & Murt, H. A. (1982). Impact of anti-smoking campaigns on smoking prevalence: A cohort analysis. *Journal of Public Health Policy, 3*(4), 374-390.

Warner, K. E., & Slade, J. (1992). Low tar, high toll. *American Journal of Public Health, 82,* 17-18.

Watson, W. P., & Little, H. J. (1999). Prolonged effects of chronic ethanol treatment on responses to repeated nicotine administration: Interactions with environmental cues. *Neuropharmacology, 38,* 587-595.

West, R. J., & Evans, D. A. (1986). Lifestyle changes in long-term survivors of acute myocardial infarction. *Journal of Epidemiology and Community Health, 40,* 103-109.

Wetter, D. W., Fiore, M. C., Gritz, E. R., Lando, H. A., Stitzer, M. L., Hasselblad, V., & Baker, T. B. (1998). The Agency for Health Care Policy and Research Smoking Cessation Clinical Practice Guideline: Findings and implications for psychologists. *American Psychologist, 53,* 657-669.

Wichelow, M. J., Golding, J. F., & Treasure, F. P. (1988). Comparison of some dietary habits of smokers and non-smokers. *British Journal of Addiction, 83,* 295-304.

Wiencke, J. K., Thurston, S. W., Kelsey, K. T., Varkonyi, A., Wain, J. C., Mark, E. J., & Christiani, D. C. (1999). Early age at smoking initiation and tobacco carcinogen DNA damage in the lung. *Journal of the National Cancer Institute, 91*(7), 614-619.

Wilbert, J. (1987). *Tobacco and shamanism in South America.* New Haven, CT: Yale University Press.

Williamson, D. F., Madans, J., Anda, R. F., Kleinman, J. C., Giovino, G. A., & Byers, T. (1991). Smoking cessation and severity of weight gain in a national cohort. *New England Journal of Medicine, 324,* 739-745.

Wilson, C. (2000, May 24). *Cigarette makers acknowledge risk* [Associated Press wire story].

Windsor, R. A., Boyd, N. R., & Orleans, C. T. (1998). A meta-evaluation of smoking cessation intervention research among pregnant women: Improving the science and art. *Health Education Research, 13,* 419-438.

Wingo, P. A., Ries, L. A. G., Giovino, G. A., Miller, D. S., Rosenberg, H. M., Shopland, D. R., Thun, M. J., & Edwards, B. K. (1999). Annual report to the nation on the status of cancer, 1973-1996, with a special section on lung cancer and tobacco smoking. *Journal of the National Cancer Institute, 91*(8), 675-690.

World Bank. (1993). *World development report 1993—Investing in health.* New York: Oxford University Press.

World Bank. (1999). *Curbing the epidemic: Governments and the economics of tobacco control.* Washington, DC: Author.

World Health Organization. (1957). *Expert committee on addiction-producing drugs* (Technical Report Series No. 116). Geneva, Switzerland: Author.

World Health Organization. (1964). *Evaluation of dependence-producing drugs* (Technical Report Series No. 287). Geneva, Switzerland: Author.

World Health Organization. (1992). *The ICD-10 classification of mental and behavioral disorders.* Geneva, Switzerland: Author.

World Health Organization. (1996). *Tobacco alert—The tobacco epidemic: A global public health emergency.* Geneva, Switzerland: Author.

World Health Organization. (1999). *Tobacco-health fact sheet* (No. 221). Retrieved January 2, 2001, from the World Wide Web: www.who.int/inffs/en/fact221.html

Wynder, E. L. (1997). Tobacco as a cause of lung cancer: Some reflections. *American Journal of Epidemiology, 146,* 687-694.

World Health Organization. (2000). Advancing knowledge on regulating tobacco products. *Tobacco Control, 9,* 224-226.

Wynder, E. L., & Graham, E. (1950). Tobacco smoking as a possible etiologic factor in bronchiogenic carcinoma: A study of 684 proven cases. *Journal of the American Medical Association, 143,* 329-336.

Young, W. W. (1916). *The story of the cigarette.* New York: Appleton.

Author Index

Subject Index

Abstinence, 59, 61, 80, 123
Acceptance patterns, 25-26
    Anti-Cigarette League, 27
    cessation movement, 38-39
    social influence in, 27-28, 28 (table)
Addiction, 8, 9
    biobehavioral framework and, 79-81
    control in, 81-82
    criteria for, 82-83, 85 (table)
    environmental factors in, 80
    evidence of, 83-85, 85 (table)
    habituating drugs, 82
    historic accounts of, 19-20, 24
    marketing approaches and, 156
    mortality risk and, 88
    nicotine exposure and, 58-60, 73
    policy coordination, 153-154
    progression to, 69 (table)
    reinforcement mechanisms and, 60-61, 73-75, 86
    severity of, 87-90
    spiritual beliefs and, 21
    terminology, 90, 91-92 (table)
    theory/evidence development, 83-85, 85 (table)
    tobacco products and, 78-79, 129
    withdrawal symptoms, 85-87, 87 (table)
Addiction Research Center in Baltimore, 101
Addiction Research Foundation of Ontario, 77
Addiction Research Foundation in Toronto, 101
Adolescent tobacco use, 66-68, 69 (table), 70, 71, 89
    multiple drug use and, 96-98, 97-99 (figures)
    sequential drug use, 102-104
Advertising, 28, 134
    limits on, 70
    marketing, regulation of, 154-156
    product placement, 67
    themes in, 66-67, 110-111
    youth tobacco use and, 67-68
Agency for Health Care Policy and Research (AHCPR), 130, 131
Alcohol, 9, 82, 88-89
    See also Biobehavioral syndrome
American Cancer Society, 38, 118, 119

About the Authors

Lynn T. Kozlowski, Ph.D., is professor and head of the Department of Biobehavioral Health, College of Health and Human Development, at Pennsylvania State University. Before moving to Penn State, he was Head of Behavioral Research on Tobacco Use at the Addiction Research Foundation of Ontario and Professor of Preventive Medicine and of Psychology at the University of Toronto. He has published widely on cigarette smoking and nicotine addiction. He has written chapters for surgeons general's reports and National Cancer Institute Monographs. He was a member of an expert committee for the Royal Society of Canada and has consulted for Health and Welfare Canada, the Canadian Cancer Society, the Ontario Heart and Stroke Foundation, and the Canadian Public Health Association. In the United States, he has advised the Centers for Disease Control and Prevention, the Food and Drug Administration, the Federal Trade Commission, the National Cancer Institute, and the National Institute on Drug Abuse. He is an assistant editor of *Addiction.*

Jack E. Henningfield, Ph.D., is associate professor of Behavioral Biology in the Department of Psychiatry and Behavioral Sciences at the Johns Hopkins University School of Medicine in Baltimore. He is also vice president for Research and Health Policy at Pinney Associates in Bethesda, Maryland, where he consults on a wide variety of issues related to drug addiction treatment, prevention, policy, and medications development. He took a leading role on tobacco and nicotine issues at the National Institute on Drug Abuse where he was serving as chief of Clinical Pharmacology when he retired in 1996. He has published research on the effects of a wide range of psychoactive drugs on animals and humans. He has contributed to numerous reports of the U.S. surgeon general on the health consequences of tobacco use, assisted the Food and Drug Administration in its tobacco regulations, and serves as an expert adviser to the U.S. Centers for Disease Control and Prevention, the World Health Organization, European Union, and other agencies concerning the science of tobacco addiction and its prevention and treatment.

Janet Brigham, Ph.D., is a research psychologist for SRI International in Menlo Park, California. The author of *Dying to Quit: Why We Smoke and How We Stop* (1998), she has studied substance abuse for more than a decade. In Baltimore, Maryland, she investigated tobacco dependence as a postdoctoral fellow at the Johns Hopkins University School of Medicine and was a fellow at the Addiction Research Center of the National Institute on Drug Abuse. She was project director on tobacco dependence treatment studies at the University of Pittsburgh, where she also did brainwave research into substance abuse etiology. A former journalist and editor, she worked for the Associated Press and for several newspapers and magazines. She has been a consultant to the World Health Organization on tobacco dependence issues. For three years, she has been editor of the quarterly newsletter of the Society for Research on Nicotine and Tobacco. Her present research interests include studying the use of multiple forms of tobacco and devising computerized testing.